MW00878011

Why is Grandma Screaming?

A Practical Guide to Improving Quality of Life in Long Term Care

Barbara F. Speedling

Copyright © 2014 Authored By Barbara F. Speedling
All rights reserved.

ISBN: 1499543476
ISBN 13: 9781499543476

For all those who have lost their voice.

Acknowledgments

I have crossed paths with many good and caring people over the course of my career in long-term care. There are countless healthcare professionals who have contributed to my education and growth, and for that I am forever grateful.

My perspective on person-centered care began to take shape early in my career thanks to the influence of two wonderful nurses, Florence Rose, RN and Martha Sweet, RN. Mrs. Rose taught me a great deal about analyzing human behavior. We worked together in one of my first nursing homes in Ohio. She treated her residents with the utmost respect and consideration and they responded in kind. The simplest of approaches could move mountains.

Martha Sweet would tell you that she hired me off the bus. I interviewed with Martha for an Activity Director's position at the nursing home in which she was the Administrator on my first day in New York City in 1986. She hired me and, as they say, "the rest is history."

It was Martha's ability to balance quality care and the business of caring with intelligence and grace that has had a lasting impact on me. She taught me that maintaining an environment of care that speaks to both the quality of the care and the quality of life afforded those receiving the care is easy if you do it every day and expect everyone else to do the same.

At a time when activity programs were rarely recognized as therapy, Barbara Nodiff, RN, took an interest in my work. Barbara was the quality assurance consultant for the nursing home I was working in at the time. Like me, she recognized the need for better education in caring for people with dementia and hired me to provide activities consultation to some of her client facilities.

Over the next twelve years, she taught me a great deal about regulatory compliance and quality assurance. It is because of her guidance that I am well-versed in regulation and effective policy development. Barbara's support of my work and generosity in exposing me to so many opportunities for growth has proven an invaluable contribution to my career. For that, there are not enough words to express my thanks.

This work would not have been completed without the friendship and shared vision of my colleagues who have contributed their thoughts to this conversation on quality of life. Thank you to Phyllis Bianco, MPA, JD, LNHA, Dr. Albert Riddle, MD, CMD, Lisa Venditti, R.Ph, FASCP, Terrence Hicks, OTR/L and Patricia Brown, RN, for helping bring this story to life.

Thank you to my mom and dad for my compassion for others and for my education. I have my sisters to thank for many things, but most of all for their friendship. A special thanks to Sr. Harriet Ann, wherever she may be, for making me do all of that public speaking in the seventh and eighth grade.

Barbara

Foreword

"You're not a nurse!" When I first met Barbara Speedling twenty years ago, she was a professional ahead of her time. At that point in her career, Barbara had been hired by a long-term care consulting firm comprised exclusively of nurse consultants up until that point. The firm's founder wanted Barbara to bring her unique background and perspective to their nursing home clients, where complaints of "behavior" were on the rise. It was clear that nursing home staff needed education in managing behaviors, but there didn't seem to be anyone we knew who had a true expertise in the area. Then we met Barbara, and everything changed.

Barbara didn't march through the nursing units with a clipboard, creating lists and lists of things we more or less already knew. Instead, she sat down with our team members and listened. She came to us as a human being, interested in improving the quality of life of our residents, and she did this by first building a rapport with our staff. She established herself as a colleague and guide and not as an auditor, which helped the staff communicate their real concerns and frustrations without fear of being judged.

The suggestions, programs, and staff training that followed reflect the years of professional and personal experience Barbara has had working and being in the company of dependent people. Barbara taught us that much of the behavior we were seeing was normal for the person exhibiting it and that *we* were the ones who had to change. For example, instead of constantly telling a resident to "go back to bed" in the middle of the night, why aren't we strolling along with them and having a conversation until they are ready to go back to bed on their own? Why are we forcing people to do anything they don't want to do? As simple as this sounds it just wasn't understood by everyone back then.

Barbara has essentially blazed a path through the uncharted waters of behavior management, and on her own, she has pioneered several behavior management programs and teaching tools that previously didn't exist in the world of long-term care.

Today's long-term care culture change movement, which emphasizes person-centered care, provides the long overdue recognition that Barbara never received from long ago colleagues and co-workers. Her interest then, as it is now, is in what motivates individual behavior. She is a true humanist with the goal of helping long-term care facilities deliver exactly what the movement teaches: person-centered care to each resident, regardless of diagnosis and level of dependence.

"Why is Grandma Screaming?" is an insightful work and a must read for anyone who works with or lives with a dependent person. She will bring you into her world back in Ohio, caring for people who would otherwise not have been treated as human beings, right through her professional career, where she was once dismissed because "she is not a nurse," to today, where her expertise is sought throughout the country.

Barbara shows us how predictable, and yes, "normal," resident behavior actually is, once you understand what motivates it. The experiences she shares from working with dependent people are deeply insightful and often humorous, but more often than not, they are heartbreaking and infuriating. She reminds us that, but for the grace of whatever higher power you believe in, "Every day without a helmet paintbrush is a good day." And in "A Day in the Life of a Nursing Home Resident," she conveys the sad but true life of a real nursing home resident that any one of us would find so dreadful we'd elope at the first opportunity if we could. We'd exhibit "behavior," too, if we were expected to spend a day like that.

Barbara thoughtfully lays out the simple but profound fact that people want what they had and shows how predictable and even logical "behavior" is when what they had is no more. Wouldn't any one of us mourn the loss of what we once had? Wouldn't we, too, be angry, depressed, or even violent by the constant reminder of our dependency?

Barbara not only brings a new understanding to her readers, but she inspires us to do better - to be better. She shows us that though we cannot perform the impossible, or turn back time, we can and should bring only our best self to the task and to expect the same of our colleagues. Caring for dependent people in a group context is not just a job. It can be done only by those who are willing to follow the Golden Rule: caring for others as you would want to be cared for.

Barbara asked me once, "How do I ensure quality?" At Victoria Home, we have successfully achieved a CMS Five-Star rating. Maintaining this rating requires constant vigilance and comprehensive buy-in from all levels of staff. But how exactly do we ensure it? There are the audits and observations and resident interviews, yes.

But how else do we do it? How are we different? Barbara always felt that we were different because we were willing to invest in staff education, and we were willing to think outside the box and implement her ideas on behavior management.

Since I always did tend to march to the beat of my own drummer, Victoria Home, where I have been executive director for the past twenty-four years, has benefitted greatly by Barbara's experience and wisdom. I didn't care back then that she wasn't a nurse. I care even less now. For me, Barbara's suggestions made common sense. Our staff felt listened to. They were given sound education and actual approaches to try when faced with difficult situations and the results we achieved were impressive. My staff and I have her to thank for the many quality programs and innovative ideas we've implemented over the years that began with a single resident-centered conversation.

While there are many good quality assurance activities going on at any one time in any quality long-term care facility, the most important, in my view, is establishing "person-centered care" as the guiding principle and culture of the facility and tolerating nothing less than the Golden Rule from each and every person on the team. Though it isn't a panacea, it's a solid foundation from which to base the rest of your programs. And having Barbara Speedling as a colleague, friend, and advisor also doesn't hurt.

Phyllis A. Bianco, MPA, JD, LNHA
Executive Director
Victoria Home, Ossining, NY
September 3, 2013

Introduction

Whether you believe in destiny or practice a defined faith, it's hard to deny that there has been an order to my life. I have always had people with special needs in my life. Often, they have been part of my close circle of friends and acquaintances.

My education has come naturally through intimate contact with people who are dependent on others for one reason or another. I've read volumes on dementia and mental illness, on wellness and person-centered care, but I've lived the experiences and revelations I will be sharing with you. It has been through that life experience that I've developed what I now believe is a keener sense of human need when circumstances are complicated by dependence.

There was the girl with Down syndrome who lived next door to my grandmother in Flushing, the boy in kindergarten who had a disorder that caused his head to grow three times the normal size, the girls in my new elementary school in Ohio—a blind girl and a girl with a prosthetic leg, the daughter of my parents' friends, who was hearing impaired, the Vietnam veteran who returned to high school as a double amputee—he later fought for the right to swim in the public pool at the apartment complex in which he lived, as some of his neighbors found it disturbing to see him swimming in the pool and others were opposed to sharing a pool with him; I suppose they thought amputations were contagious.

There were the countless young, disabled students I met and became friends with in college. There were the special needs children I transported every day as a school bus driver in my twenties, learning behavior management on a trial and error basis as I struggled to manage these kids with no training or experience. There are countless others I've met and come to know through my work in long-term care. Some I've chosen to tell you about because they have helped shape my knowledge and understanding of what quality of life is really all about.

I was a nursing assistant in a nursing home in Ohio for a day and a half in 1973. No certification was required for this work at that time, so my orientation consisted of being instructed on how to take vital signs and then a facility tour by the Assistant Director of Nursing.

It was during that tour that I had my first taste of *behavior*. Dinner was being passed to residents in their rooms as we walked through one of the nursing units. Just as we approached the next room, a dinner tray flew out into the hallway, crashing to the floor, the contents splattering against the wall.

My tour guide laughed uncomfortably saying, "I guess Mr. Smith doesn't like his dinner." She then whispered something to another nurse, and we continued on. I asked if she knew why he reacted so violently rather than just asking for something else, and she said she didn't know, that he "just does that."

My first day on the job was interesting, albeit a little disgusting, as I tried to keep a very large, comatose woman with a bad case of diarrhea clean, dry, and comfortable. I found another of my residents lying on the floor in her room. She'd obviously fallen out of bed. I had not been instructed on what to do in this situation, but the other aide I asked said I should put her back in bed.

As I went to help her up, I couldn't help but inhale the strong aroma of awful body odor, coupled with the smell of a fresh bowel movement. I was thinking that someone hadn't helped this lady bathe lately. I was also thinking that this was not exactly what I'd envisioned when I signed on for this job. I thought I'd be delivering iced tea and cookies to little grandmas and grandpas, not be elbow deep in feces and fighting back dry heaves.

I returned the second day to try again. I am, after all, a sensitive soul and thought long and hard about how much these folks needed help. If I could do some good and bring some happiness to these people, a little discomfort was a small price to pay. That day, however, I was assigned to a fortyish young man who had a diagnosis of multiple sclerosis. The disease had robbed him of full use of his hands, and he needed help with all of his personal care.

He rang his call bell, and I responded, greeting him and asking what he needed. He told me he had to urinate and asked that I place his penis in the urinal and hold it for him while he relieved himself. I was mortified! I had never considered that I'd have to handle a strange man's penis. I couldn't imagine doing that. I apologized to him, started to cry, and explained that I just couldn't possibly do that, that I was sorry, but that I just couldn't.

I quit that job that afternoon and went to work in fast food. I decided that was a service I could provide without too many surprises. I would find out that not only was I wrong about the surprises part, but that it definitely required the same kind of maturity and customer service perspective of treating the other guy the way you'd like to be treated as being a caregiver does. It's all about being sensitive to the customer's needs.

That experience was nursing assistant boot camp at its best. That's what usually happens to the new kid on the block in the nursing home world and probably in most care environments. Give the least experienced the toughest or least liked residents to take care of and then watch what happens!

I've learned after these many years that this is a standard indoctrination process for new certified nursing aides (CNAs) in many nursing homes. Depending on who's minding the store and the culture of the caregiver pool, this borders on being abusive to both the inexperienced caregiver and the resident.

In many cases, real abuse does occur as a result of poor training and the lack of maturity of the staff, including the middle management staff. These are the first-line supervisory folks who are generally promoted because they are good at their particular job but not necessarily because they are the most mature or effective managers.

It is in the design of the environment of care, in the depth and consideration for the needs of the population served, and a vision that demands each individual be recognized for his or her specific, unique history and set of circumstances that the goal of lasting, quality care is achieved and sustained. This will apply across all levels and types of care.

More importantly, it is the shared mission and vision of those who care that will be the foundation for a truly satisfying, person-centered approach to care and treatment. Overcoming the obstacles of human-ness, office politics, and despair over the lack of resources and support is the challenge to leadership.

Wanting to assist in achieving that goal and actively pursuing bet-ter understanding and avenues of improved care is the personal chal-lenge. Do you care enough to effect real change? Are you committed enough to shrug off being ostracized for caring too much or being seen as a Pollyanna or a drama queen?

In more than thirty years of caring and teaching, being seen as a Pollyanna has only increased the interest others have in my work. People say I think *differently* and marvel that I've been able to maintain my perspective and my empathy over the years. How could I not?

While on assignment at a facility dedicated to the care of people with traumatic brain injury, I had the opportunity to observe a most amazing young man. I would watch him make his way down the hall from the elevator to the art studio, slowly inching forward one push of his chin against the plate that operated his motorized wheelchair at a time. More than ten minutes elapsed before he reached his destina-tion after traveling a distance of less than fifty yards.

Once in the studio, I saw the instructor fit him with a large helmet that had a paintbrush attached to the forehead. The instructor loaded the paint reservoir with paint and then positioned the young man to enable him to paint on this large canvas.

He began moving his head to the extent possible, slowly making a pattern of lines and spots on the canvas. He signaled to the instructor some time later that he needed a new color, and the process began again.

Paralyzed with limited movement of his head, this brave, creative, sensitive man continued to find pleasure and purpose in creating these beautiful, abstract paintings. When I returned home, I had several postcard-sized prints of his and other residents' paintings framed in a collage that hangs at the foot of my bed.

Each morning, I'm reminded that every day without a helmet paintbrush is a good day. That my life is good, that I have more just by being independent and able to survive on my own than any of the people I may cross paths with in my work that day. That I have no reason and no right in the presence of those who long for the simple freedoms that I have to complain about providing the care and service I signed on to provide.

If I no longer want to abide by that commitment, I am free to leave. I am free to take my lack of commitment, my lack of consideration, and my failure to treat others as I'd like to be treated and leave these folks to the care of someone better than me.

Caregivers do not have the right to visit their discontent on those who depend on them for care, safety, comfort, and consideration. In spite of all of the political and consumer attention paid to national initiatives for improved care and intensified regulatory oversight, there are still gross injustices visited on these populations every day that go unrecognized and unresolved.

As you'll read later, I spent my college years as a driver and attendant for an accessible transportation service on campus. It was no coincidence that I would receive this bonus education while at Kent State University studying music. It was through this life experience, this indirect education that I have formed my thinking on quality of life and on what little it takes to improve life for the dependent.

What I hope you will take away from this writing is that there are simple, practical ways to approach the holistic care of individuals. Where there is a genuine interest in the population to be served and a commitment to care well, there is the potential to create truly meaningful, satisfying lives regardless of medical, intellectual, or other psychosocial challenges. It costs nothing to pay more attention to detail.

one

Quality of Life

Quality of life is one of those intangible concepts interpreted differently by every individual. Where some may define the quality of their life in terms of how much money they have, others will find value in what they have left as a legacy to future generations.

If you have autonomy and choice, the criteria for quality of life are endless. You may find pleasure and satisfaction in traveling, exploring new cultures and cuisines, joining a community theater group, doing extreme sports, searching for antique treasures, playing the violin, or meeting new people.

There is something to look forward to in the planning of your excursions and the things you will pursue for pleasure. There is excitement, anticipation, and an elevation in mood that may endure long after the adventure has ended. You feel alive.

If you are dependent and living in a structured setting, controlled by others and unable to access the things you need to sustain your quality of life, the criteria shrink. The smallest of pleasures become paramount. Your personality and the way in which you respond to simple, everyday situations may also be drastically different than if you were well and living independently.

Making sure you have a clean towel for your shower in the morning so that your aide won't have to use a sheet or paper towels to dry you after bathing. Towels are in short supply. Stealing the dinner roll off your tablemate's plate because the evening snack you're supposed to receive is never offered and you get hungry. With a cold plate dinner being served at 4:30 p.m., you're ravenous late in the evening. The cupboard is usually bare, except for some graham crackers and warm apple juice. I'll pass.

Many of the moods and behaviors demonstrated by cognizant, institutionalized people can often be traced back to common, everyday triggers that you or I might have a similar reaction to: noise, being told *no* in response to something you want to do, having to sit among strangers all day with whom you have nothing in common and whose behavior is often offensive or annoying to you, or being spoken to harshly, or handled roughly in response to a request for the assistance you are supposed to be receiving. You might feel sad, angry, disappointed, militant, sarcastic, vengeful, overlooked, or depressed in response to any number of situations institutionalized people experience on a daily basis.

Complicate common reactions with a diagnosis of Alzheimer's disease, mental illness, brain injury, or developmental disability, and the difficulty in understanding and resolving issues of mood and behavior becomes an even bigger challenge. Losses in memory, reasoning, language, motor function, vision, hearing, and speech require that the analysis of the triggers to these moods and behaviors be substantial and evaluated from the perspective of how diagnosis, personality, and what Dr. Riddle refers to as "baggage" impacts perception, comprehension, and response.

Further complicate the equation by removing all productivity, purpose, and satisfaction from the life of the dependent person. Contribute a healthy dose of boredom and a lack of consideration for their needs, and you have an emotional ticking time bomb on your hands. Extreme emotional response will only be controlled, stifled, or sedated for so long.

A Day in the Life of a Nursing Home Resident

5:30 a.m.	*I'm awakened by night shift staff for breakfast that is served at 7:30 a.m.*
6:45 a.m.	*I'm seated in my wheelchair along the corridor in my "parking space" as staff arrives for the day shift, carrying large cups of steaming, hot coffee from the local coffee boutique. The aroma makes me want to jump out of my chair and grab it from their hands. I love coffee! I can't speak, so I scream as they walk by.*
7:45 a.m.	*My breakfast is late, cold, and not satisfying. The coffee is barely more than colored water, and they don't stock half-and-half. It's skim milk or nothing. Ick! The room is noisy and crowded, awful music is playing on the radio, and several of my tablemates have improved efficiency by eating breakfast and moving their bowels all at the same time.*
8:15 a.m.	*I'm sitting in the dining room amid my pungent tablemates, waiting for my turn to go to the bathroom. I'm thinking they should let me go first since it's quite apparent they've already done so.*
8:45 a.m.	*I'm sitting in the dining room, waiting for the activity to begin.*
10:00 a.m.	*The activity leader arrives, places all of us in a large circle, and takes out a big ball. For the next twenty minutes or so, we toss the ball to each other to the accompaniment of marching band music. Then it's over, and the leader leaves.*
10:30 a.m.	*I'm sitting in the dining room waiting for lunch to begin. The TV is on some obnoxious talk show, my neighbor across the way is taking her clothes off, the man next to me is picking his nose, and somewhere behind me, two women are fighting over who owns the book they both want.*
12:15 p.m.	*Lunch arrives. Chicken, again.*
12:25 p.m.	*I'm sitting in the dining room listening to the staff gossip and talk about how much they hate this place. I'm wondering if their rising emotion is having any impact on the way the staff member at the next table is shoving the spoonful of food in that lady's mouth?*

12:35 p.m.   *I'm waiting to go to the bathroom and for the next activity to begin.*

2:30 p.m.   *Today's activity program is cancelled—more sitting until dinner and then bed!*

3:15 p.m.   *A song I used to love to sing is played in the dayroom, and it reminds me of all I've lost. I try to leave the room because I don't want to hear it, but the staff won't let me, so I kick at them. I don't want to be reminded of who I will never be again, but they don't know that, they don't really know me, and they don't care. Later, I get a new pill that silences me and makes it difficult for me to kick at them when they provoke me with their ignorance.*

Satisfaction and Productivity

I've always felt that life is pretty much over when you stop moving forward. Without dreams, aspirations, and crazy notions of what might be, what joy is there in living? With no opportunity to plan, to anticipate, no opportunity to ride the wave of mounting excitement over the coming of something you've been waiting for, or working toward, or hoping upon hope to experience before you die, what's the fun in living?

Those who are in the business of providing care and support to the dependent fail to recognize the importance of having goals beyond moving your bowels at least every three days. If you are being treated in the short-term following a health crisis expected to resolve itself with proper care and treatment, your goal to regain your physical well-being and return home represents your entire quality of life at that point in time. It's something to work toward, to look forward to.

If you are admitted to an institutional environment for the long haul, however, your entire quality of life becomes focused on the basics: being clean, dry, well fed, and pain and annoyance free. After the initial indoctrination period, most residents' criteria for quality of life become small and focused: having a single room (usually out of reach for most nursing home residents), to be able to shower daily and use the toilet in privacy, to have the chance to win money instead of silly prizes at bingo (so you always have soda money), and to be treated considerately and respectfully by those who are there to provide the care and support you require.

In my numerous quality of life interviews with residents of nursing homes, assisted living facilities, adult homes, residential group homes, and those served by adult daycare centers, it is the small, almost insignificant things that define quality of life and satisfaction. Simply put: *people want what they had.*

Let's think about that. What they *had.* What do you have now that you would lose in moving to an institutional environment? How would those losses impact your mood and behavior? I'll use my own life as an example:

1. I currently enjoy a home in which I have complete privacy and control. My response to losing that privacy and control would likely manifest in sarcasm, escalating impatience and agitation, and certainly a resistance to being controlled.
2. I love to drive my car and find driving to be a soothing, meditative activity, particularly highway driving. It also represents a type of freedom that cannot be replaced. My response to losing my car, my freedom, and this favored, stress-reducing activity will likely be more than a little agitation and restlessness. I think it will be my biggest loss.
3. Noise is the most significant annoyance in my life. I do not like a noisy environment and do everything I can to control my sensory input. My response to the constant noise experienced in institutional living would be more of the same impatience but with a little screaming to be heard over the din.

I could go on, but you get the idea. In just those few examples, the losses are great and have little to do with tangible *stuff.* The loss of independence is tragic. It has been devastating to every dependent person I've ever interviewed.

Do they *adjust?* Some do, some never do and never will. Some find their quality of life in becoming a constant annoyance to the people they perceive as "holding him in this prison," as one man I met put it.

So, what is our responsibility as caregivers? In my mind, the mission is clear and simple: care for others as you would want to be cared for. Yes, that's right, the Golden Rule. The simplest of concepts captures the core intent of all of the person-centered care philosophies.

Put yourself in the bed, in the wheelchair, at the dinner table next to the man who spits his food out on your plate, or in the shower, where the hot water runs out just as you get naked, wet, and soapy. Consider your reactions, your behavior, in the aftermath of the violence that occurs because the part-time caregiver assigned to you tonight is poorly trained and has an attitude.

Now, how do you feel? How would you react in these various scenarios? Might you get angry, use foul language, or raise your hand to someone if you felt frustrated, threatened, or offended? If you had dementia or some other emotional or intellectual disability, might your interpretation of everything be inaccurate and your reactions intensified? Would you lose all shred of control when forced to defecate in your diaper because the caregiver assigned to care for you left the building for dinner, and no one else will assist you because you're "not theirs?"

Would the caregiver responding to your mood and behavior understand all the motivations behind what they see? Do they know enough about you as an individual, about your personality, your rituals, routines, and idiosyncrasies, your coping skills, and about the impact of your illness and circumstance to know what causes these extreme emotions and what calms them?

The Dying Man: I was reviewing the grievance process in a nursing home when I was told that one particular resident was a "big problem." Staff reported that he was difficult, refusing medication and care, not wanting to get out of bed, and generally dissatisfied with the care he received. He rang the call bell a lot, too.

When I asked them why he was so disgruntled, the response was a collective, "Don't know. That's just the way he is." The recreation progress notes said that he planned his own day and was pursuing the things he liked to do. From these descriptions, I expected to find a rather outspoken, defiant man, busy in his room doing what he liked to do.

This was not the case.

The man I saw lying twisted uncomfortably in his bed was dying. It wasn't even necessary to know the nature of his illness. You could just see that he was dying. You could see the bones in his arms and in his chest. He was wasting. He was dying.

I introduced myself and asked if I could talk with him. He looked at me with wide eyes, then shrugged, and said, "I guess." He'd been watching a television show that he now turned back to. The TV was on the nightstand, which was to the left of the head of his bed. In order to see it, he had to turn on his side and hold the side rail with his right hand to be able to remain in that position. He was weak.

Looking around the room, it was cluttered and not as clean as it could be. There was a bureau against the wall at the foot of his bed. I asked if he had considered having the TV on top of the bureau. He had no remote and no money to buy one. There was no one who could purchase one for him, either. He was alone.

His family had given up on him a long time ago because of the way he was living his life. Trouble and gang mischief, drugs, alcohol, and questionable partners had led him down a precarious path.

There were several previously opened bottles of soda on the shelf in his closet, and the door to the closet was missing. He said he kept them there because it was difficult to get something to drink because the staff was very busy. I pointed out that it was warm and probably flat. He knew, but it was better than nothing.

The pitcher at his bedside that he used as a cup had the remnants of brown liquid in it. I wanted to think it was soda, but I'm not sure that it wasn't just dirty water. There were flies in the room. They buzzed around him, and he slowly swatted at them. Did he tell anyone about the flies? He didn't think it would do any good.

He closed his eyes and sighed deeply. He talked about the terrible bouts of diarrhea he'd had. He rang the call bell when he felt it coming. "You can feel it in your stomach, you know, that gurgling." He tried to ring it in time, before he soiled himself and the bed. "I hate for them to have to clean me up. They don't like it when I mess up the bed." They never come in time, he explained.

He talked about his pain. His legs were long, maybe just a little longer than the bed. He couldn't walk far by himself, and even shorter distances lately. His legs ached. He was dying. Do you receive pain medication? Tylenol, when he asked for it.

As I was ready to leave, he told me that he knew he did this to himself, that his lifestyle and his choices robbed him of his health and of his life. He asked, "Do you think they (the caregivers) know, too? Is that why they feel the way they do about me? Why they ignore me?"

I'd like to think that this was just an unfortunate, isolated case of caregivers who had lost their perspective. I'm sorry to say that it is not. It is common. It is at the root of what is wrong with our institutions.

I left this man wondering why no one had stopped to think about how someone who is dying might behave. If you were dying, would you be angry or bitter or defiant or just plain miserable? Might your family and friends say you were difficult to understand or difficult to deal with? Would they assume it's just *you*, or would they understand that it was your grief, your depression, your disappointment, fear, and anxiety over your impending death that was talking?

What has happened to our perspective on human need and human emotion? And if we have lost our perspective on what the dying need, how can we create a livable community for those who have a life yet to live?

When I approached the staff caring for this man and explained what I'd learned about him and his "behavior," the general response was that there wasn't enough time to give him that kind of personal attention. Some said they would like to, but there's just too much work to do and not enough staff. Sadly, that is too often a true statement.

They would respond now to my findings by giving him a lot of attention, finding him a better bed, cleaning his room, getting him something to drink, and resolving his TV remote issues. As long as

I was his "squeaky wheel," he would experience improved customer service. The trouble is it often isn't sustainable.

I find that the vast majority of professional caregivers are genuinely concerned about the people they are caring for. It is often the lack of resources needed to provide quality care to an increasingly diverse and complex population that weighs heavily on even the best of caregivers. Over time, whole environments become overwhelmed, complacent, and jaded.

There will never be enough staff to provide the kind of individualized, person-centered care we idealize, but there could certainly be more than what you will find in the majority of long-term care facilities. The government has established minimum staffing standards for certain positions; however, many essential categories of direct care staff that contribute significantly to a person's quality of life are not included. Two prime examples are CNAs and activity leaders.

The number of CNAs is determined by the facility and generally based on the number of total beds and the acuity of the care being provided. The general ratio of staff to resident for CNAs on a forty-bed unit is somewhere between eight to twelve/CNA on the day shift, thirteen to fifteen/CNA on the evening shift, and twenty plus/CNA on the night shift.

The average ratio of activity leaders to residents in a 200-bed nursing home is forty or fifty to one. A staff of four or five full-time activity leaders will be responsible for programming that occurs seven days a week, including evenings, weekends, and holidays. With this kind of staffing there is little meaningful, satisfying activity going on.

Federal and state staffing regulations mandate "sufficient" staffing. Without established guidelines, however, facility owners are allowed to decide what is "sufficient." Sadly, the definition of what is sufficient is often determined by budget and not by care needs. Moreover, the decision-makers are rarely clinical professionals. There is no requirement for owners or administrators of long-term care service organizations to have a clinical background.

In today's long-term care environment, we hear a lot of terms like culture change, person-centered, and individualized care bantered about. With scarce resources and no realistic hope of additional resources in the foreseeable future, human or otherwise, successfully achieving and sustaining a quality existence for those living in long-term care environments is all about *thinking differently.*

two

What Is Quality of Life?

Kent State

I had the good fortune to spend most of my college days at Kent State University in Ohio. I was majoring in vocal music and aspired, as many did, to be rich and famous. To pay the bills along the way, I learned to drive a bus. It was a time when women were just beginning to venture into new areas of work historically dominated by men. I reasoned that it would be a good skill to fall back on should it take me some time to reach fame and fortune.

It was also to be the most valuable education and training I could have asked for in planning for the future. The experiences I had left a lasting impression on my thinking about how to care for another human being. The role that these experiences and my skills in music and the arts would play in my life and my career years later didn't become clear until long after my time at Kent.

It was the mid-1970s and awareness of the needs of the disabled and dependent was just beginning to emerge on the national agenda. Nursing homes were still regarded as "poor houses," reserved for those who had no alternatives for care. The Medicaid fraud and abuse scandals of the late 1970s motivated sweeping changes in the long-term care industry.

The Americans with Disabilities Act (ADA) didn't become law until 1990, making Kent State a leader among universities in ensuring accessibility to the disabled. The campus offered accessible dormitories, a program in which students could work as attendants to their disabled peers and an extensive transportation service that provided access to both campus and off-campus destinations. The town of Kent was also disability-friendly, being among the first cities to install curb cuts throughout the city to make life easier for the disabled.

The Campus Bus Service, a university owned and operated transportation service, was staffed exclusively by students. Several alumni functioned in the administrative and management roles. Not only did it offer the best wages on campus, but it was a lot like belonging to a fraternity. CBS provided daily and charter service to the university, the town of Kent, and surrounding towns as far north as Cleveland. Charter service was also available to national destinations.

As staff, we were exceptionally well trained in safety and the special considerations for disabled students. Our training included how to manage a manual or motorized wheelchair, manipulate it up and down stairs, disassemble and reassemble the parts, check the battery on motorized chairs, manage turning corners in the van without throwing the passengers out of their seats, and other technical information that ensured we were more than competent to carry this precious cargo.

What I learned from the more seasoned drivers was more about how to manage the mood and behavior of that precious cargo. Since this was a service provided to the public, there were no rules beyond driving safely and getting you to your destination. This was my first introduction, albeit a poor one, to behavior modification.

Instructions from one senior driver for responding to the rude behavior of one frequent rider: "If the mouthy, profane passenger refuses to cease and desist, deliver him to his destination, but once there, turn off the battery to his chair until he apologizes. If he refuses to apologize and refrain from future abuse of the drivers and passengers, tell him you will leave him there on the curb, powerless." The driver went on to say that he always apologizes rather than be stranded and is less offensive "for a while, anyway."

What stays with me about those years and all the people I met is how they found their quality of life in spite of tragic and dire circumstances. Faced with what many would consider insurmountable odds, those brave, motivated, happy people taught me that there is always something good to be experienced every day, no matter the challenges, the sadness, or the pain. There is always life where there is hope.

The People
The College Years

T rode my bus on the Campus Loop route every morning. He'd get on around seven thirty at the stop in front of McGilvrey Hall carrying a donut for me and his brown bag lunch. He'd greet me with, "Good morning, Mrs. Bus Driver," peeling the donut, which was icing-side down in the palm of his hand, from his hand and offering it to me. I'd thank him, take the donut, and put it aside in a napkin for later.

T lived at a group home not far from campus. He worked in the kitchen at a hospital in the next town. His job was everything to him. In spite of his developmental disabilities, he was proud of his work and his contribution to the lives of the patients and staff being serviced by the hospital kitchen.

His morning bus rides were more than just a way to get to work. Riding the bus allowed him to mingle with students, faculty, staff, and visitors to the college as just another guy on his way to work. He would talk with students sitting near him, asking what they were reading or where they were from. I think this interaction made him feel less "special" and contributed greatly to his feelings of confidence and self-esteem.

Working at the hospital defined him. It was who he was. One day, he boarded the bus with a look of distress on his face and a newspaper pressed firmly against the back of his white uniform pants. He climbed the stairs, no donut, and didn't greet me. He quickly sat down on the newspaper in his usual seat across the aisle from me, but he didn't look at me or anyone. He simply stared at the floor with a look of panic and confusion.

There was a strong odor of feces now that the doors were closed. I knew it was coming from him. I asked him if he was OK. Without looking up, he said, "I couldn't help it. I have new pills, and they gave me diarrhea. I couldn't help it, I shit on myself." Yes, that was evident.

I suggested he get off the bus and go back home since he wasn't feeling well. He became immediately upset and anxious, saying he had to go to work, no matter what. They were depending on him. He then proceeded to recite the instructions he must have been given in orientation about lateness and sick calls. He knew his coworkers depended on him.

His job, his responsibility, and the fact that someone was depending on him made his life purposeful. His quality of life was defined by his job and the social networking the commute and the work he did allowed him.

On a later pass through campus, *T* was again on my bus. Apparently, the supervisor at the hospital told him to go home until he felt better. He was glad that he had gone to work and fulfilled his responsibility but relieved that he was allowed to go home without penalty or damage to his good reputation.

❧

A was a young woman in her mid-twenties who described herself to me as a perpetual student. She had a disability that left her dwarfed with no ability to hold her head up without assistance.

One of the things I remember most about her was her weekly trip to the midnight showing of the *Rocky Horror Picture Show*. With a roll of toilet paper in hand, she'd head to the show dressed as Dr. Scott. She knew the dialogue by heart and always came prepared to participate.

Like many of the disabled students on campus, *A* had attendants who helped her with her daily care needs. Most were young, good looking guys who were attracted to this free-spirited, confident, fun-loving, young woman. They were able to look past her disability to see who she was, and that was something I found fascinating.

One of her attendants attached a board to the back of her wheelchair to support her head and keep it upright. He later began using a red bandana to secure her head to the board to improve her position-ing. Being the '70s, this was both functional and fashionable.

Driving *A* to class one morning, I hit a bump, and her head fell out of the bandana. I looked in the rearview mirror to see her chin to chest. I apologized and said I'd pull over to reposition her.

"No! Keep going. I want to get to class!" she yelled. "When you make the next turn, turn hard, and I'll be OK." I did as she said, mak-ing a hard right turn at the next intersection, and her head found its way back, resting against the board until we reached her destination, and I was able to readjust the bandana.

She later explained that she wanted to get to class early so she would be able to sit next to this guy she liked. It was a large lecture hall, and if she was late, she'd lose her spot. Then she rolled her big, brown eyes, and making a "Woo hoo!" sound, said he was the best thing about this lecture class!

❧❧

D had a baby face, freckles, and piercing, blue eyes. He couldn't speak. His disability had robbed him of his speech, so he communicated by writing on his notepad or with gestures. He was always smiling.

As we got to know each other, we developed another level of com-munication that was based on familiarity. I knew his routine, the things he liked and didn't like about school, about being dependent—I'd observed him over time, watching his reactions to certain things, things people said or did.

He was proud and fiercely independent. Even when his ambula-tion deteriorated to needing two canes, he wouldn't accept help get-ting up if he fell. He would do it, thank you very much.

We remained friends throughout our college years. After gradu-ation, we settled in towns not far from each other. He had landed a job in his field, found an apartment after being turned away by many who did not want the liability of a disabled tenant, and got his driver's license.

He came to visit me a couple of times, and it was always nice to see him. Then he invited me to his home. Sitting on the couch in his living room one afternoon discussing his décor, he leaned in and started to kiss me.

I'd never expected that! I'd never thought of him that way. I pulled back, explaining that I didn't feel that way about him. The look on his face was a mixture of confusion, embarrassment, and disbelief, and then the look of disgust and disappointment I'd seen him show people who'd offended him.

He leaned back, sizing me up, looking away, shaking his head, and then looking back at me. He made a loud sound and waved his hand at me, as if to say, "What the hell!?" Then he grabbed his notepad and began to write.

He was confused and angry. He didn't understand, and he thought I liked him. He wrote that I had always been nice to him. He thought the attention I paid him in school was special, that I went out of my way to be nice to him and be his friend. Because I'd held his hand or hugged him, he thought I was attracted to him.

I never knew his feelings went so deep or that he'd misunderstood my friendship as more than what it was. I think now it was my own immaturity that caused me to overlook how my affection and attention toward him appeared to him. His compromised ability to delve into conversation and really express himself over the years complicated everything.

If I had been less naïve, I would have recognized that there was a whole lot of thinking and passion going on inside this young man who aspired to be a journalist. It was my own ignorance that let me believe there wasn't more to him.

A few weeks after that visit, he wrote to me. He let me have it. I would never again underestimate his thinking. I never saw him again. I've thought about him many times over the years. I think about how I hurt him because I was inexperienced and insensitive.

❧

J was one of several young men I'd met who was paralyzed as a result of breaking his neck in a diving accident. In his case, he dove into a pond late at night after drinking with his friends and hit bottom, leaving him paralyzed from the neck down. After a time and with intense physical therapy, he was able to operate an adapted, motorized wheelchair with his head.

He would describe his memory of his accident, often chuckling about how he couldn't believe he'd actually survived. I'd wonder how he could think this was funny at all!

Lying on the bottom of the pond, he realized he couldn't move and wondered if his friends would find him before he died. The next thing he remembered was being in the hospital, his mother crying and feeling as though his body was gone, even though he could see it. "That was really weird, man, you know?"

J had a girlfriend who also worked for the transportation service. She and I were often scheduled on the same van. We talked a lot about their relationship and what it felt like to be with someone you had to do everything for, including bladder and bowel care.

It didn't faze her. She loved him. She could see past the wheelchair and the disability to the bright, witty, charming, young man who always had a joke to tell and who lived a happy life in spite of his challenges.

૭ેન્જી

M was walking to lunch one day in downtown Cleveland when he was struck by a stray bullet. It left him completely paralyzed from the neck down. He was completely dependent. Unlike *J*, he was never able to afford a motorized chair, so he had to rely on someone pushing him everywhere.

When he'd tell the story—and the brain injury he sustained as a result of the shooting caused him to forget that he'd told you already, but you didn't interrupt him out of respect—he would always tell you he wasn't angry about it, but that he wondered, *why him?* Even when it frustrated him, he took it in stride.

He said he knew there was nothing he could do about it now, that there was no way to turn back time, that there was nothing and no one to be angry about—they never found out where the bullet came from—but that he wonders what his life would have been like had he done something different on that day?

Going to college distracted him from his never-ending replay and analysis of his accident and the resulting sadness over the life it's left him. He liked being engaged, learning, growing, and making friends. He had a gentle, thoughtful way about him and a sad but genuine smile.

⸒⸑

B was paraplegic as a result of a motorcycle accident. He had been a member of some kind of bad boy motorcycle club and had a blowout at a high speed one day. He was not the nicest of people and had a real knack for catching me off guard with his explosive impatience. If you didn't move fast enough, you just might suffer a whack with the metal clasp of his seatbelt.

He liked hitting you and getting you to react and give him a reason to do it again, only harder this time. He was angry that his life of crime, mischief, and abuse of others had been interrupted, so he was adapting those skills to his new situation.

He only hit me once. The first time I picked him up. He called me names, teased me for being overweight, and generally did whatever he could to get a rise out of me.

Fortunately, he was not the first bully I'd encountered, and I used a skill I'd perfected in high school to diffuse the situation. Find the common bond, the place where your brains and hearts meet on how it feels to be disappointed, unable to move as you'd like along your path to satisfaction. Validate each other's sadness. It changes things.

I ignored his comments long enough to engage him in a conversation about his accident. I opened with a story I'd heard recently from another passenger about his injury—he'd fallen two years ago while skiing and sustained a spinal cord injury that left him paralyzed from the waist down. He had told me he plans to learn to ski again, that it's possible with adapted equipment. He was eager to get back on the slopes.

I said I didn't know if I could be that resilient. I remember thinking he was very brave and that I would not have the courage to ski again. *B* immediately responded with how he was going to ride a motorcycle again, too. He said he'd seen a story on television about how people like him ride horses, sky dive, and all kinds of things you might think they can't do anymore. He wasn't going to allow a little paralysis to keep him off his Harley!

I had read him correctly. He had a big ego and considered himself tough, a man's man, not afraid of anyone, or anything. I don't think he really thought about riding a motorcycle again until I told him that story, but he would never admit that.

He went on to talk about why he loved riding and why he missed it. He said it made him feel free, powerful, and wild! He bragged about fast his bike was, the tricks he could do, and how he rebelled against wearing a helmet.

His expression changed. I think he was reminded of how the speed, the tricks, and riding without a helmet contributed to his current status. That opened the door to a brief comment about his feelings on now being dependent—he didn't like it, it made him feel frustrated and angry. It was that frustration and anger that fueled his offensive behavior.

He closed the door quickly that time, but there were a number of conversations that followed that I believe helped him see what could still be, in spite of his disability. I introduced him to the skier who invited him to join the wheelchair basketball team on campus. Some months later, he told me he'd taken a ride in a friend's sidecar, and he was back on the road!

I don't want to give the impression that I tamed him, but I was able to help him open a door. All of that frustration and anger began to dissipate as he became more involved in living his life. He was able to channel his emotions in a more productive way, naturally diffusing his need to be abusive to other people.

❧❧

R was a handsome, engaging, young man diagnosed with a progressive, neuromuscular disorder. He had big, brown eyes, a bright, winning smile, and a deep, velvety voice that could make anyone melt.

He was a humanities major, concerned with life and people. He aspired to make the world a better place for people like himself. His illness left him with weakened muscles and diminished ability to do the simplest of things. He had no strength to grasp things with his hand and had trouble operating the joystick on his motorized wheelchair. He talked of designing a better mode of transportation, futuristic images involving robots and computerized operating systems.

We had an instant chemistry. I thought he was adorable, smart, funny, certainly nice to look at, and he had these wonderful, creative ideas of what could be. I remember thinking more than once that I hoped he'd have the time to accomplish his dreams. People diagnosed with his particular illness didn't generally live long lives.

I thought about him a lot in the summer of 2012. I didn't know why he was on my mind so many years later. I searched for him on the Internet and found a photograph of him. He was smiling that winning smile and looking good after all those years.

I was excited to find him and eagerly followed the photograph link. I was thinking we might get to connect and share stories about where life had taken us. The photograph link I followed took me to an obituary written earlier that summer by his staff at the transit organization he'd eventually joined after college. He had lived a relatively long and happy life. He had lived his dreams. I think he wanted me to know that, and that's why he was in my thoughts that summer.

The Nursing Home Years

I have my sister, Gail, to thank for my lengthy and satisfying career in long-term care. I was working for the local school system as a school bus driver at the time. Out of college for a short time and uncertain about what my education would lead to in terms of a viable occupation, my sister encouraged me to respond to an ad for an Assistant Director of Activities in a local nursing home.

I had no idea what the job entailed, but Gail was certain that my music and arts background would make me a desirable candidate. I landed the job and quickly saw what she meant when she said it was ideal for me. My skills were well-suited to the position, and I excelled quickly, achieving my certification in therapeutic activity and moving on to become the Director of Activities at another facility.

The next facility provided both pediatric and adult long-term care services. I had not anticipated seeing children as young as three in a nursing home, but there they were. Considering how long they might live in that nursing home, quality of life, purpose, and satisfaction took on a whole new significance.

For the first time, I realized that a nursing home was not exclusive to the old and frail. In fact, there were children—young children— who would spend their entire lives in a building like this. Many of the adults were also younger than I'd anticipated—in their fifties and sixties—and had a long history of institutionalization as a result of mental illness, functional, or intellectual disability.

In fact, many of them had lived together in a state psychiatric facility, so they had known each other for some time. They were like a family in the way they supported and protected each other. As I came to know them, I could see how their attachment to each other and their growing love of the children that resided in the facility afforded them a purpose, a focus to their day.

Unlike the frail elderly, these residents all had lives yet to live. Some were robbed of their life because the parents, teachers, and medical professionals of the time didn't know how to manage their disability. J spent his life in the state facility because he was deaf. That was it. He was deaf.

Tall and lanky, he would position himself at the front door of the facility, greeting visitors and helping other residents in and out. He liked opening doors for people, delivering mail, and helping out on the pediatric unit. It gave him purpose and satisfaction. It also helped him overcome what he'd been told and came to believe over the years that being deaf was equal to being stupid.

I had no real knowledge or understanding of mental illness or intellectual disability at that time. There were many residents whose behavior I didn't understand. There were also some who frightened me with their outbursts and unpredictable behavior.

C introduced himself to me on my first day at the facility. He stood at the base of the ramp leading to the front door asking me, "Hey, lady, are you new here?" I said I was, and he asked the same question a few more times as he made his way up the ramp. I thought he was going to shake my hand, but, instead, he slapped me in the face!

I didn't know how to respond. I was startled and unsure of what to do. He looked at me, tucked his hands behind him, and said, "You are new here, yup, new here, new here..." As he walked away, I wondered what that was all about.

As I grew to know him, I saw that his pleasure seemed to come from upsetting others. He never hit me again, but he tested the waters with many others. He would often make derogatory remarks under his breath about other residents or staff, would do things to annoy others deliberately, and he enjoyed creating whatever tension and chaos he could. He would then stand back and enjoy the fray.

L and *F* were lovers. They'd lived together for many years in the state hospital. *L* was a large, gray-haired woman who walked with a sort of "bobbing" gait. Other residents looked up to her. Always with her pocketbook and short, white socks, *L* was the leader of the pack.

F had the look of a prize fighter, with his crooked nose and hunched, faux boxing stance when you greeted him. He liked to come off as gruff and unfriendly, but as you came to know him, you saw a softer side. He loved *L* and looked out for her. She ordered him around, and he complained, but their devotion to one another was plain to see.

E was a twenty-eight-year-old man with an intellectual disability. He was tall, thin, and walked with his knees bent, as if he were about to stop and kneel. He was never without his navy cap pulled down low over his eyes. He always referred to himself in the third person— "*E* is funny, isn't he?" And he loved to smoke.

You could find him most days sitting in the lobby, legs crossed, and fingers positioned at his lips as if he were smoking, but he had no cigarette. Passersby would be queried, "Do you have a weed for *E*?" He'd then go on to say to himself, "*E* needs a weed. Do you have a weed? A weed is good. He likes it, yes, he does."

Conversation was tough and always focused on smoking. I tried to engage him in conversation and various activities, but he was always distracted by his desire to smoke. So, I began talking to him about smoking. I was a smoker at the time and, sometimes, we would smoke together. I asked him once why he liked to smoke and, rather than respond, he just looked at me. It might have been the first time we actually made eye contact.

After a few moments, he turned away, took a long drag off of his cigarette, and said, "It's pretty. It's good. He likes it. It makes him pretty. Yeah, ha, ha, ha, he's pretty. He is a pretty boy." I agreed, saying I thought he was great. He then said, "Yes, he's great. *E* is great."

Then, I asked him about his family, and he responded to a question for the first time. He used similar words to describe his family— pretty, good, and now, great. Our conversations continued over time, and his vocabulary for responding to questions began to grow. He made eye contact more often and was able to respond more directly in conversation.

He remained obsessed with smoking and focused his conversation on his favorite pastime. He was, however, more social and more easily engaged as he was challenged more often intellectually.

I learned later that he had lived at home for many years in virtual isolation from the world. His parents were loving, but uncomfortable with his disability and unwilling to institutionalize him as a child. As he got older, it became more difficult for his parents to care for him, so placement was inevitable. He'd lived first in the state psychiatric hospital and was later transferred to this nursing home.

By the time he was admitted to the facility, he had very little exposure to the world and very little interaction with people outside of his family. The lack of intellectual stimulation had left him lost for words and unfamiliar with the art of social conversation. As his skills and vocabulary grew, so did his comfort and ability to be social and communicative.

Many of the residents at that facility went out to school or to sheltered workshops during the day. There was a pervasive understanding among the long-term care community that being involved and having a purpose was essential to quality of life. Those who remained in the facility were afforded meaningful activity that was designed to accommodate not only their interests but their skills and abilities.

I was fortunate to work with a group of professionals at that time who understood that creating a quality life for children and adults who are dependent is no small task. Looking back, I was surrounded by smart, motivated, caring people who recognized all those years ago what "culture change" really means. My understanding of what quality care and quality of life really are grew in the years I spent there.

I moved back to New York in the mid-1980s and continued to work as a activities professional. Unlike what I'd experienced in Ohio, where purpose and involvement were recognized as essential, I learned very quickly that many facilities overlooked the importance of meaningful activity and social involvement. As long as some music was playing and the daily bingo game was running, all was right with the world.

People perceived my job as easy, something anyone could do. It was classically described as game playing or party time, yet I saw it differently based on what I'd learned in the early days of my career and in those precious years at Kent State.

Early on, I began to challenge the idea of what meaningful activity was. I didn't see the benefit of merely entertaining people or understand how it was OK to pacify those who couldn't participate in what was going on by parking them in front of a television or playing music that had no particular impact on them.

Using the sheltered workshop model I'd learned about in Ohio, I began to develop a different approach to meaningful activity and quality of life. My focus was on the individual's life experience, occupation, and personality.

The activities I began to develop for people were reminiscent of their life in some way. The activity either replicated an occupational, social, or domestic activity they continued to show interest in or something tailored to their current level of understanding and skill.

Activities in the latter category were generally sorting, matching, or counting activities that could be easily accomplished with instruction and oversight. For example, I might have someone shine a shoe or separate buttons by size. In the end, it was the accomplishment of a purposeful task that brought about the satisfaction.

I continue to teach this model, believing that challenging people intellectually and functionally is far more beneficial to their mental and spiritual health than merely entertaining them. Moreover, occupying people in purposeful activity is preferable to forcing them to sit idly for hours on end waiting for something good or interesting to happen.

The most important thing I've learned from the individuals I've introduced you to thus far is that you have to really know and understand someone before you can help them live a quality existence. Consider the epidemic numbers of people in long-term care diagnosed with Alzheimer's disease or a related dementia. The experts tell us that the most meaningful, therapeutic intervention for this population is reminiscence. There is comfort in the familiar.

If this is true, then the most significant component of person-centered care is the holistic assessment of the individual. It is through this holistic assessment process that we learn the keys to distinguishing between symptoms of illness, reactions to situations and circumstances, and personality. Moreover, it's the first step in recognizing what will constitute a quality existence for the individual. Person-centered care in the truest sense.

three

Assessment

ANTIPSYCHOTIC DRUGS CALLED
HAZARDOUS FOR THE ELDERLY

"Nearly one in seven elderly nursing home residents, nearly all of them
with dementia, are given powerful, atypical, antipsychotic drugs, even
though the medicines increase the risks of death and are not approved for
such treatments, a government audit found...Risperdal, Zyprexa, Seroquel,
Abilify, and Geodon are 'potentially lethal' to many of the patients."
—*Gardiner Harris, NY Times, Published: May 9, 2011*

The use of psychotropic medication in long-term care is common in
the management of behavior. Medication is generally the preferred
response to challenging mood and behavior because it's quick, requires
little actual thought or work, and makes the behavior stop—sometimes.

If it doesn't work, we add more or a little of another drug or a stat
dose of something to knock the resident out until we can find another
drug that might work. What results in most cases is a mess created out
of ignorance and, in some cases, a lack of interest or concern.

The holistic assessment process must begin with a method of validating the person's diagnosis. Alzheimer's disease, for example, is only
distinguishable from other neurodegenerative diseases upon autopsy.[1]

---

[1] 2013 Alzheimer's Association Facts and Figures

A diagnosis of mental illness or brain injury requires specific diagnostic testing to achieve an accurate diagnosis, as well.

According to the Alzheimer's Association, it is important for a physician to determine the cause of memory loss or other symptoms. Some dementia-like symptoms can be reversed if they are caused by treatable conditions, such as depression, drug interaction, thyroid problems, excess use of alcohol, or certain vitamin deficiencies.[2]

If diagnostic information is not provided by the referral source, requesting that information will be important to developing the plan of care. In some cases, the receiving facility may want to develop an admitting protocol that includes specific steps to rule out conditions that may resolve over time, such as malnutrition, dehydration, or cognitive issues caused by improper use of medication.

Once the diagnosis is confirmed, staff education should follow. Every effort should be made to prepare the caregiver team for the person they will be caring for. A person's diagnosis should be known and the common symptoms discussed.

Knowing as much as possible about how a disease process will impact a person's actions and reactions will be the first step to distinguishing symptoms from behaviors. For example, helping the caregiver to understand the impact of a diagnosis of paranoia on a new resident's ability to adjust to change may prevent them from doing something to trigger paranoid behavior.

For example, unpacking the personal belongings of this new resident without permission and without the new resident being present is sure to cause friction and, in some cases, may trigger a violent outburst or altercation with the offending caregiver. Most of which, based on what occurs in many environments, will be blamed on the new resident and labeled a "behavior."

Had the caregiver been properly prepared for receiving a new resident with mental health challenges, one of which is paranoid thinking, the caregiver might have anticipated the negative reaction and gone about the task of unpacking with the new resident. In this scenario, the

---

[2] http://www.alz.org/mnnd/documents/10signs_physicanfactsheet_final.pdf

cause of the resident's reaction is the caregiver's actions. Not providing adequate education and information to caregivers could be interpreted as a form of abuse, both for the resident and the caregiver.

Creative solutions require not only good education but interest and a commitment to be flexible and tenacious. You must be willing to work at finding the most effective solution to any problem. Where it involves the care and treatment of human beings, you have to take it a step further. You have to also be able to empathize, to see the world through the other person's eyes, if you want to achieve the greatest quality of life for everyone you care for.

To be able to empathize, you have to first know the person. A holistic assessment of the *person* should look next at personality, lifestyle, occupation, and education, as well as clinical needs. Knowing who the person is and where they've been and how they've responded to the peaks and valleys in their life will tell you a great deal about the kind of clinical care they require and the responses to that care that you might anticipate.

The Waif: I am asked to help the care team address the mood and behavior of a young woman who is causing major issues in their facility.

She is forty-one and paralyzed, except for some minimal movement in the right hand she uses to control her motorized wheelchair. Admitted two years ago, known to staff as a "hell raiser," mouthy, offensive to everyone, abusive to her elderly and disabled neighbors, off-color most of the time, never happy, never satisfied, has her friends smuggle marijuana into the facility—a trouble maker.

Social workers and recreation therapists have provided support and encouragement. They have counseled her on her inappropriate behavior and offered her adapted crafts and music to entertain her. They have given in on her demand for a private room after she abused every roommate they attempted to pair her with. She is unappreciative of their efforts.

It was reported that she and one of her visiting friends used the craft materials to make an obscene poster for her room. In another report, she is said to have spit at her social worker who she describes as a "goody-two-shoes"—"She doesn't fucking get it...she's a baby, probably never been laid. That's what she needs, to get laid. I was eleven the first time I got laid, and I loved it!" She turns her attention to the male housekeeper working nearby. "I'd like to get laid, how 'bout you?"

Psychiatry and psychology are called in. She refuses to see either one—"I am *not* fucking crazy! They're fucking crazy!" They attempt to quiet her with medication, but she refuses to take it. No one knows what else to do.

Her social history is sketchy according to the staff. No one knows much about her. The social worker's admission assessment reflects very little information, except that she was homeless before the accident that paralyzed her at twenty-one. When I asked what kind of accident, the general consensus was that it must have been a motor vehicle accident. She won't talk about it.

When I attempt to interview her, she refuses. I tell her I want to understand why she is so angry and work with her and the staff to resolve whatever is fueling her anger. She laughs at me and calls me stupid. She says, "The staff don't care about what I think or what I want. I want to get the fuck out of here, that's what I want. That's what they could do for me." She tells me to get out and shut the door.

I looked at the original admission documents sent from the hospital two years earlier, and it was there that I learned her story. Born to a drug-addicted mother who made her living as a prostitute, she was molested more than once by her mother's customers at a young age, turned out as a child prostitute at eleven, abandoned at thirteen, and homeless for most of her teens.

She lived in shelters or on the street. There was information about an aunt who had agreed to let her live with her when she was fifteen, but it didn't work out, and she returned to the streets. She made her living through prostitution, drug sales, and stealing.

At twenty-one, she finds herself in a hotel room with a john who has a fragile ego and a temper - often not a good combination. They've been drinking and drugging most of the night. He later tells the police officer who arrests him that she started laughing at him when he couldn't get an erection, so he started punching her in the face. When that didn't stop her from laughing, he shot her seven times.

And they wonder where the anger and defiance, the depression, the disappointment, the filthy mouth, the mission to make everyone else as miserable as she is comes from?

Long-term care environments are increasingly diverse. Young people, aging people, physically or intellectually disabled people, mentally ill people, and epidemic numbers of people with Alzheimer's disease or a related dementia are living together in environments that are not designed well for the broad range of needs these populations present. There has been little thought given to how these diverse customers will find individual satisfaction in a one-size-fits-all environment.

The Importance of Distinguishing between Symptoms, Reactions, and Personalities

Alice bursts into the Administrator's office red-faced and panting. "Please, mister, I have to talk to you! Please, it's important. I have to talk to you now!" She pauses for a moment and then begins her plea again, only louder and quicker this time. "Pleeaasse! I have to talk to you now, mister! Pleeeeaaasseee!"

She begins to bob in place, leaning on her rolling walker decorated with a multitude of ribbons, bows, flags, and other assorted memorabilia she's collected over time as she is asking him to *please, please, please* talk to her.

She goes on without waiting to be invited to tell her tale of the dress that was promised to her by her cousin that has never arrived. Can he call her cousin and find out if she's sending the dress? Can he ask her if she can't send the dress if she can send some money so Alice could buy her own dress? Can he make the social worker talk to her because she always says she's busy and closes the door in Alice's face? Can she have a drink of water because her throat is dry and she feels dizzy and her heart is pounding in her chest and she thinks she might be having a heart attack because her father had a heart attack and she looks just like her father...

The Administrator is not a clinician, he is a businessman. He doesn't understand bipolar disorder or recognize that he is looking at someone who is unable to control her mounting anxiety and mania without appropriate treatment. He doesn't know that the common side effects of the medications she is receiving to treat her bipolar disorder—Depakote and Seroquel—are often headache or other increased body pain and discomfort, increased nervousness, feelings of dizziness, or fatigue.

These potential side effects in combination with the known symptoms of bipolar mania cause Alice to be unable to wait, unable to control her impulsive behavior, and need for immediate attention. In other words, this is not *behavior*, but the manifestation of symptoms and reactions to treatments that may need to be evaluated and modified to achieve the desired remedy and improved quality of life for the individual affected by the illness.

Because he doesn't understand what he is looking at, the Administrator responds to Alice in a way that only serves to escalate her anxiety. He tells her he's busy, and he'll talk to her later. He then suggests she go to the activity that's being offered in the dining room or to the social worker's office.

Alice explodes in an even louder, more pathetic rant about how no one likes her, how the social worker doesn't talk to her, how the other residents tell her to shut up at the activity programs, how she must find out about the money her cousin was sending because she needs a new dress, and she thinks she's having a heart attack and begins to sob loudly, uncontrollably, holding her chest and looking as though she is going to faint. She manages a weakened, almost hushed "Pleeeeassse, mister, pleeaaaaaassseee" in a final attempt to win his support.

Education on mental illness and how to recognize the symptoms of diseases like bipolar disorder is lacking in most long-term care environments. The long-term care industry has given little attention to ensuring caregivers are properly trained in psychiatric care due to the outdated perception that adult residential communities and nursing homes are unaffected by mental illness.

Younger and more complex populations are common in these environments. Often impacted by traumatic brain injury, long-standing psychiatric illness or other psychosocial challenges like substance abuse or homelessness, this atypical population presents new and different challenges in behavioral health.

The epidemic numbers of people with Alzheimer's disease or a related dementia has been recognized in long-term care as worthy of more than casual attention. Federal regulations require a minimum of annual education in dementia, with some states requiring more classroom hours than others. There is no specific regulatory guidance, however, for education in mental illness or intellectual and developmental disabilities. It is left to the individual provider to decide what is necessary. The only exception would be in facilities where additional, specialized education is required due to the type of population served (i.e., people with traumatic brain injury) or a specialized service provided. The education requirements will differ by state, as well.

According to an article published by the National Institutes of Health in 2010, over the past decade, the proportion of new nursing home admissions with mental illness other than dementia, including major depression and serious mental illness, such as schizophrenia and other psychotic disorders, *has overtaken the proportion with dementia only.*[3]

Understanding Dementia

Dementia is a progressive state of mental decline, especially of memory function and judgment, often accompanied by disorientation and disintegration of the personality. Alzheimer's disease is the most common form of dementia; however, dementia is the result of many other conditions and disease processes, including Parkinson's disease, AIDS, traumatic brain injury, stroke, vascular disease, and chronic alcohol or substance abuse.

---

[3] Grabowski, Aschbrenner, Rome and Bartels, "Quality of Mental Health Care for Nursing Home Residents: A Literature Review," *National Institutes for Health*, 2010.

Dementia comes on gradually, eventually robbing the person of all ability to function intellectually. Family caregivers often report subtle, early signs of memory loss, like misplacing a set of keys or forgetting to pay a bill. As the disease progresses, it impacts every aspect of communication and ability to remain independent in day-to-day living.

According to the 2013 Alzheimer's Association's Facts and Figures, every sixty-eight seconds, someone in the United States develops Alzheimer's. By midcentury, someone in the United States will develop the disease every thirty-three seconds.[4] Add to these staggering statistics the growing diversity of the long-term care environment, and the need to ensure a caregiver workforce that is well-informed and equipped to create and sustain a quality living environment becomes clear.

The symptoms associated with dementia are complicated and often misunderstood by caregivers as "behavior." A comprehensive assessment must scrutinize not only medical issues but delve into personality, life history, social and occupational experience, and the individual's thoughts and feelings about a variety of things lost to dependency. More importantly, the history of how this person has adapted to his or her life over time and how he or she has traditionally behaved in times of stress or extreme emotion must be explored.

Dr. Albert Riddle, MD, CMD, has been a colleague and friend for many years. In essence, we've grown up together in long-term care, often overlapping in client facilities and working together on various education and quality improvement projects.

Over the last few years, Dr. Riddle and I have blended our skills in behavioral health into a comprehensive program designed to sustain an environment of care focused on wellness and meeting the holistic needs of each resident. Through an expanded perspective on what fuels wellness and satisfaction in people who are dependent on others, we have developed an approach that looks not only at physical or functional rehabilitation, but true, person-centered, therapeutic intervention for those with wounded bodies and broken spirits.

---

[4] 2013 Alzheimer's Association Facts and Figures.

In the following passage, Dr. Riddle discusses how personality and reactions develop, followed by an examination of how aging and disability, coupled with our personal baggage, impact mood and behavior:

Formation of Personality Traits

As we go through the stages of cognitive development, we have the concurrent formation of our personality. This process is influenced by a combination of genetics, culture, environment, and memory of life experiences. Our personality, once developed, has the ability to color and place a framework around future life experiences, thereby making each one of us unique.

We are all familiar, to some extent, with the famous work of Sigmund Freud that seems to tell us that sex is the major driving force behind everything. Freud gave us the concept of the id, ego, and superego, the three components that work together to form personality.

Probably the most cited theories in psychology were given to us by Jean Piaget, who wrote the book Genetic Epidemiology. He suggested that children have experiences that allow them to build unique databases that expand over time. As time passes, they are able to sort their knowledge into groupings called schemes.

As new knowledge is acquired, it may be assimilated into existing schemes, or the new knowledge may trigger revision of an existing scheme or may require formation of an entirely new scheme. He theorized that personality was developed over the course of four distinct phases—sensorimotor, preoperational, concrete operational, and formal operational.

Development of Behaviors

Many of the behaviors that we see in the elderly are a product of their personality in combination with a breakdown in cognition. We deal with situations throughout our lives that threaten us or make us unhappy, anxious, or uncertain.

We adjust to those situations by building a library of coping mechanisms.

Through trial and error, over time, we learn what works best for us. With experience, these coping mechanisms that we have developed and fine-tuned over time become almost instinctual.

We accumulate baggage over time, as well. Within that bag are our successes, our failures, our losses of family, friends, health, property, and autonomy, our sources of pride, our sources of shame, and beyond that, the skeletons in our closet.

As a physician who recognizes the value of a holistic assessment, Dr. Riddle understands the importance of addressing not only the symptoms of a person's illness but the baggage that will complicate the person's care. It is that baggage that will influence the person's reactions and interactions in the environment. Without a solid understanding of both the illness and the individual, person-centered care will remain an unreachable ideal.

If you are going to care well for someone and create a meaningful existence, you must know them. Beyond understanding a medical diagnosis, distinguishing between what is a symptom and what is a reaction or attributable to personality is essential to understanding that individual and who he/she was before the onset of his or her disability. With that knowledge, the framework for developing a quality existence for that individual will be clearer.

The impact of comorbidities like mental illness, traumatic brain injury, or intellectual disability will further complicate behaviors and reactions. The failure of many long-term care facilities to provide their staff with education and training on these subjects further deteriorates the quality of life for people who are dependent.

Without proper education and training in these disease processes, abuse, neglect, and mistreatment abound. In a 2002 article on mental health services in long-term care, the following challenges to the development of non-pharmacological interventions to address behavior were cited:

- Observational studies of nursing assistants indicate that they fulfill primarily a custodial function and have limited interactions with residents.
- Nursing assistants often have negative feelings when residents show aggressive behavior.
- They tend to avoid residents who are verbally or physically aggressive.
- The cultural and ethnic background of the nursing home staff may influence their perceptions of problem behaviors and non-pharmacologic interventions.
- A wide variance in the ability of individual caregivers to tolerate aggression.
- Staff members may hesitate to replace medications with non-pharmacologic interventions if they anticipate that this practice may lead to more disruptive behavior and add to their workload.
- They often see the sedating effects of psychotropic drugs as desirable and might prefer their use to resident activity.[5]

In addition to these factors, there are significant systemic issues that impede the delivery of quality, person-centered care. In my experience as a consultant to long-term care environments, the following additional common challenges exist:

- Diagnosis is not always known or accurate at the time of admission screening;
- Staff education and training in caring for people with special needs is lacking;
- Staff lack basic understanding of disease process and the ability to recognize symptoms;
- Assessments often fail to explore personality and lifestyle, two important factors impacting the person's perception of and reactions to the environment;

---

[5] *Psychiatry Services* Cody et al. 53 (11): 1402. Marisue Cody, PhD, RN; Cornelia Beck, PhD, RN; Bonnie L. Svarstad, PhD.

- Communication between disciplines is weak in tracking behavioral patterns;
- Care teams are weak in understanding and applying behavior modification; and
- Medication is the often the preferred intervention because it is quick and requires little staff involvement.

Pharmacist Lisa Venditti, R.Ph, FASCP, is another of my longtime friends and colleagues I credit with educating me over the years. We have always shared a knack for looking differently at the possible remedies a resident is offered. As consultants, we have been witness to a host of circumstances whose negative outcome could have been avoided if they had been handled differently.

A case I worked on some years ago involved a medication error that ended in the death of a nursing home resident. A telephone order for a medication the resident received to treat a chronic condition was received from the physician.

Telephone orders are a common way for physicians serving nursing homes and other long-term care facilities to communicate medication and treatment orders between scheduled visits. The law in most states requires the physician to authenticate and sign the telephone order onsite within forty-eight hours.

The nurse who transcribed the telephone order into the resident's medical record made a mistake. The physician prescribed one pill, three times daily, and the nurse wrote three pills, three times daily. The responsibility to review and validate this order passes through several hands before the resident receives the medication.

In this case, the order was reviewed by the nurse who transcribed it, the pharmacy that filled it, the nurses who followed the transcriber on the next two shifts and should have questioned the new order when they signed off as having reviewed it, the nurses who administered the medication per the erroneous order, and the physician who authenticated and signed the erroneous order onsite. No one caught the error.

In the investigation that followed, three of the nurses involved blamed the error on being overwhelmed with responsibility. This happened long before the belt tightening we face today began, but not having enough hands was the primary reason for error or oversight, even then.

In the next passage, Lisa discusses two scenarios in which the use of psychoactive medication did not always produce the desired effect. She explains that it is common for caregivers to overlook simple remedies in favor of medication. In the following example, she illustrates how thinking differently opens the door to practical, non-pharmacologic intervention:

> A resident with dementia admitted to the nursing home liked to hum. She hummed the same song over and over. It was a pleasant song, actually a well-known circus theme, but day after day, hour after hour, she was driving the staff crazy.
>
> The staff asked that the resident be placed on a psychoactive medication to control her symptoms. The physician prescribed an anti-anxiety medication to calm the resident. It not only stopped the humming but quieted her completely. She was unable to walk on her own and had stopped communicating with staff and other residents.
>
> The consultant pharmacist reviewed the medication profile during her monthly review. She noted the new anti-anxiety medication had been prescribed without benefit of a psychiatric evaluation. She questioned the diagnosis of anxiety.
>
> She knew the resident well and had always known her to be a happy woman who loved to hum. She asked the staff why the medication had been prescribed and found out it was for the incessant humming.
>
> She explained to the staff that this was equal to a chemical restraint. The resident was not in any "frightful distress," which would have warranted the use of the medication that had been prescribed.
>
> She recommended the resident be offered an iPod with headphones. Different songs were loaded onto the iPod, and the resident now hummed to different songs instead of only

one. The anti-anxiety medication was discontinued and the
staff and resident were all happy.

In the next passage, she tells the story of how even medication that
is prescribed appropriately can be potentially harmful if not properly
monitored:

A woman admitted to a nursing home with a diagnosis of
mild dementia began to show signs of cognitive decline, becom-
ing more confused and resisting care. She was not receiving
any psychoactive medication at that time.

Her physician prescribed a common medication indicated
for mild to moderate dementia. Within two weeks of starting
the drug, she began to experience nightmares that caused her
to scream. She stopped eating and lost a significant amount
of weight.

These symptoms were associated with a dementia diagno-
sis, and so her physician increased the dose of the dementia
medication. He added an adjunct medication to the regimen
that was also appropriately indicated for dementia. The resi-
dent began having multiple falls that ultimately resulted in a
hip fracture.

The consultant pharmacist completed a medication regimen
review and noted that the dementia medications prescribed for
the resident had side effects of nightmares, loss of appetite, and
falls. She alerted the physician, and the medications were discon-
tinued. The resident's cognitive status improved to her baseline
state, and she began to eat and gain weight. The falls ceased.

In summary, Lisa reminds us that, "The key to avoiding these situations in the future is education." In both cases, responding to a deeper
understanding of what influences the behavior proves to be more
effective than attempting to simply stifle it. The ability of direct care
staff to evaluate behavior on this level requires not only education but
an environment that supports this kind of analysis.

Beyond the lack of staff education and training are the human factors that impact mood and behavior. Little consideration is given to how boredom and a lack of meaningful, satisfying activity impact behavior and function. Even less consideration is given to the fact that living in a controlled environment would be difficult for anyone and far more complicated for the person with dementia, mental illness, or other functional or intellectual disability.

Extreme emotion is bound to occur in the absence of understanding and consideration. Without outlets for managing extreme emotion and stress, behaviors associated with anxiety, restlessness, social unrest, and resistance to care will likely be intensified. Few environments that I have observed recognize that no one can be *fine* all the time.

What Makes People Do What They Do?

Dr. J was a retired dentist with a moderate to late stage Alzheimer's dementia. He was in his mid-eighties, physically in good shape, and pleasant enough. The only time his behavior would change was when you forgot to call him "Doctor." I had seen him completely ignore a staff member who called him by his first name, only to see him respond politely to another staff member who addressed him as Doctor.

It is not uncommon for a professional person to expect to be addressed by a title he/she has worked hard for. Nor is it uncommon for the person to respond with a sign of offense or annoyance if their status is overlooked.

Mr. D is a retired business owner with a vascular dementia who is described by the staff as someone who considers himself to be of an elite status—worldly, accomplished, and well-read. He chooses not to socialize with the other residents who he considers less capable than himself. He makes comments about the way others are dressed, how old others look in comparison to himself, and other generally offensive remarks loud enough for all to hear.

His adult children acknowledge that their father was not always easy to get along with. His daughter describes him as a perfectionist who expected his children to excel in school and in life. He put a lot of pressure on them and on himself to be the best at everything. He enjoyed being recognized as a successful person.

Several weeks into his residency, he agrees to eat his noon meal in the main dining room. He has eaten his lunch in his room until now, preferring to read rather than socialize while he ate.

He arrives in the dining room wearing his usual jacket and tie. He is seated at a table by the window and offered his choice of coffee or tea. He asks what type of tea they have and is disappointed when he learns that they only stock a generic brand of tea. "Of course," he responds sarcastically, waving a hand as if to dismiss the server. He doesn't want any tea.

Another resident arrives and seats herself across from him at the table. She is petite and neatly dressed in a floral housedress. She is wearing a large, beaded necklace and dark-rimmed eyeglasses. She smiles at him and asks his name.

Without responding to her question, he loudly asks no one in particular, "Who put this bitch at my table!?" He looks around for someone to respond, then turns his attention back to his unfortunate tablemate. "Where did you think you were going dressed like that? You're obviously in the wrong place!"

He signals for a staff member and suggests they move this woman to a more appropriate group. He references his own attire compared to the woman's and asks the staff member how someone could have possibly mistaken them for having anything in common?

Mr. D's reaction to the woman is really quite normal given what is known about him and the way he sees himself in relation to others. It is quite common for people to make judgments about others based on what they look like or to choose social companions based on commonalities and "chemistry."

The staff later described his reaction as behavior attributable to his dementia. I challenged them to consider how all of the personality traits they'd already witnessed and could easily describe contributed to the way he treated his tablemate.

In the end, we agreed that his reaction was predictable based on what was known about his personality, his ego, and how he saw himself.

Too often, personality and common, mature reactions to various social scenarios are labeled "behavior" rather than being seen as normal for the individual and only complicated by illness or disability and fading impulse control.

Consider how the environment alone contributes to the reactions of the people living there. More than half of the people are compromised by some level of dementia, suggesting that their perspective on where they are and what is happening is distorted, at best.

Imagine never really knowing where you are or who the strangers are that order you around all day. You are thinking you have to go to work and that you have a family to support. The people who are ordering you around tell you that what you think is not true. They tell you that you *are* home, even though this place looks nothing like any home you remember and that you don't work anymore.

I know few adults who would react kindly to being told to sit down or that they couldn't go outside and sit in the garden or that they couldn't go home anymore. The vast majority of people I meet in my lectures acknowledge that they would respond poorly to being told what to do by anyone. They value being in control and wouldn't respond well to someone who was challenging their autonomy.

In this next passage, Dr. Riddle discusses a common conflict between resident and caregiver that often escalates needlessly into a heated or, sometimes, violent exchange. In this example, the caregiver is focused on the task at hand—getting the resident to finish his meal—rather than on the resident's level of satisfaction with the meal and the dining environment.

> It is important to all of us to have choices. An ambulatory, independent resident of a skilled nursing facility is sitting in the dining room of the facility eating his dinner. He finished his main course, decided that he was full, and got up to go back to his room.
>
> A nursing assistant, who is feeding a dependent resident, saw him stand and noticed that he has not touched his dessert.

She said to him, "Mr. R, you are not done yet. You didn't eat your dessert." He responded, "I am finished," as he turned to leave the dining room.

The nursing assistant approached him. "Mr. R, you have not finished your dessert. Let me call the nurse to help you." Mr. R then angrily and loudly stated, "I'm not stupid, I don't need help. I hate this place. I have to get out of here and get some air, or I'm going to kill someone." He raised his walker and seemed like he was going to throw it just as the nurse, who had been called to help him, arrived.

What happened during this encounter? We have a resident who is sitting in a common eating area and has completed his meal and decides that he does not want to have dessert. We have a nursing assistant who sees that he has not finished his dessert and wants him to stay and complete his meal.

It is not clear what was motivating Mr. R to want to skip dessert and leave the dining room. Maybe he is full from consuming the main course. Perhaps he wants to remove himself from the crowded and noisy atmosphere of the dining room. It could be that there is a television program that he wants to get back to his room and watch. It really doesn't matter what his motivations were as long as they were not interfering with the rights of the other residents and was not disruptive to the ability of the staff to maintain a safe environment and provide good care.

This was a person who was making a choice, in this case choosing to skip dessert and leave the dining room. He should have been allowed that choice.

You may have wondered, as you read the scenario, why the nursing assistant didn't ask him why he wanted to leave and offered him an opportunity to have his dessert in another location, such as his room. The situation, as handled, threatened the freedom of Mr. R to make a choice and act upon it. Think of how frustrating that must have been for him, especially if there was of pattern of this in his day to day living at the facility.

The staff reviewed the incident, and a decision was made to request a psychiatric consultation for Mr. R as soon as possible. As per facility policy, the staff wrote a full report of their concerns for the psychiatrist to review when he came in to do the assessment of Mr. R. The statement that was written by the staff was as follows:

"Mr. R is easily agitated and becomes threatening. He raised his walker and threatened to toss it. He is very confused and angry. In addition, he resists care and is verbally and physically abusive. He gets especially anxious and agitated at night.

His medical history is significant for Hypertension, Dementia, Depression, Anxiety, and Diabetes Mellitus, and his medications include Paroxetine for Major Depressive Disorder and Panic, Rivastigmine and Memantine for Dementia of Alzheimer's type, and Amlodipine Hypertension."

The psychiatric assessment was conducted within a few days. No other incidents occurred from the time of the incident in the dining room to the time of the psychiatric assessment.

The psychiatrist wrote, "Male resident who has dementia with depression and a behavior disturbance. It is possible that his agitated depression may be under medicated. It is worth trying an increase in Paroxitine to 40 mg (he had been on 20 mg daily). I would also like to add Extended Release Divalproex Sodium 250 mg at bedtime. If this is not helping in two weeks, consider increasing the dose to 500 mg at bedtime. Finally, you can add Lorazepam 0.25 mg twice daily to reduce anxiety. Don't forget to check Valproic Acid levels."

What started out as someone wanting to get up and leave a room turned into a plan of care for a behavioral problem that included chemical interventions in the absence of non-chemical interventions. If we analyze this case using the ABCs of behavioral assessment, we would start with describing the behavior as a resident who became angry while trying to leave the dining room.

The antecedent event was the nursing assistant trying to stop him from leaving. The consequence of the behavior was minimal in that there was no physical injury, and though there was a brief verbal disruption in the presence of other residents, there was no threat perceived by the other residents. The staff felt threatened by how he manipulated his walker as he tried to walk away, however, he was trying to position the walker to safely ambulate and did not intend to threaten anyone with it.

If we can agree that the antecedent event was restricting his ability to make a choice and act on it, the most effective potential non-chemical intervention becomes readily apparent. First, let him leave. Second, realize the consequences of his leaving. He ate his dinner. It is not crucial that he have his dessert. Offer him the choice of letting him have it in his room or some other safe location, and if he doesn't want it, accept that.

If these measures had been followed, there would have been no disruption, there would have been no perceived need for a psychiatric consultation, and there would not have been the recommendations that followed to increase his medication load. It all seems so clear and so easy, yet, so often it doesn't work out this way.

&oc;

It is so important to understand how the individual lived and how he sees himself in relation to the world and others in it. The admission assessment should explore education, occupation, and feelings about communal living and socialization, in general. Adding the following questions to the assessment process will help the team to better anticipate certain actions and reactions and plan proactively for intervention.

- **Known or potential triggers to behavior:** For example, phobias, environmental issues (i.e., temperature, noise levels), those related to personal preference (i.e., Mrs. X prefers dresses to slacks but is unable to express this verbally. She often disrobes in response to discomfort).

- **The pre-dementia/pre-disability personality of the resident:** For example, if Mr. X was always a strong personality, taking charge, giving orders, etc., this aspect of his character will likely be evidenced. Unaware that this is "normal" behavior for this resident, staff may interpret his responses as agitated or aggressive.

- **Social and occupational history:** What type of social person was he/she? What type of work did he/she do? How did he/she feel about status, control, reputation, or "keeping up with the Joneses?" Understanding how people perceived themselves in society, both socially and occupationally, may shed some light on behaviors now being addressed.

- **Family dynamics that may be reflected in the resident's interaction with others:** For example, traumatic events (i.e., domestic violence, sexual abuse, loss of a child, etc.) that have occurred, regardless of when they occurred in the resident's life, may motivate certain behaviors. Staff may also find that bearing a resemblance to someone in the resident's past may trigger certain responses, particularly if the relationship was unhealthy. The family generally does not offer this type of personal information. Research into this area should be fully explained to the family to ensure they understand why such information is necessary.

- **Successful remedies employed by the resident in times of distress:** What methods did the person employ for self-soothing? Some people engage in sports, some take a bubble bath, some eat, some take a drink or a smoke, and still others seek out a sympathetic ear. What did this person do to decompress?

- **Preferences and routines that will serve as the foundation of individual plans:** While most of this information is reflected in the social history and MDS, knowing the resident's favorite color, song, nursery rhyme, etc., will help staff develop diversionary interventions. Families should also be encouraged to provide photographs, audio/video tapes, or other familiar items that would be used in developing diversionary activity.

The final piece to the holistic assessment process involves developing a daily existence that is meaningful and satisfying to the individual. In achieving this level of person-centered care and quality of life, the challenges currently faced in behavioral health begin to fade.

Addressed appropriately through careful assessment and personalized response, the time staff now devotes to investigating complaints, fighting with residents who are resistive to care and control and completing the reams of paperwork associated with negative events could be used in more productive ways. A little satisfaction goes a long way to deterring negative behavior and the need for medication or other, less reasonable, personalized interventions.

four

Creating a Meaningful, Satisfying Existence

As I shared with you earlier, I began my career in long-term care in therapeutic activity. I have never strayed far from those roots, always believing that having a reason to live, to get better, to be happy on any given day was what made life worth living.

V was a man in his fifties who'd sustained a brain injury as a result of a mugging shortly before arriving at the nursing home. Not long after he arrived, he left the facility unsupervised—he "eloped."

This is not an uncommon occurrence for people who are newly admitted to a nursing home or other residential setting, particularly if they have a dementia diagnosis. In some cases, there is no dementia, just an unhappy person who was not given a choice in moving to the nursing home.

There are times when the decision is made after a significant health event (i.e., stroke, fracture) by family members or community social service agencies without the participation of the individual. Many times, people will attempt to elope out of anger or defiance.

I've always thought that to be a pretty normal reaction for any adult being forced to do something he/she doesn't want to do. I don't imagine it would take me long to express my dissatisfaction by saying something like, "I'm out of here," and heading for the door. It's my personality and how I react to circumstances I find intolerable.

Some years ago, I was returning from a field trip with several residents. As the bus pulled up in front of the nursing home, one resident said she wasn't going to any nursing home and refused to get off the bus. Even in the later stages of her dementia, going to a nursing home was remembered as a bad thing.

We had to make several more trips around the neighborhood, finally convincing her to come into the building from a rear, unmarked entrance. As we rode around in an effort to diffuse her emotion, she continued to make comments about not going to a nursing home.

Like many people with dementia, she usually had difficulty expressing herself clearly. On this occasion, however, she was able to be quite clear in her agitation over thinking she was being taken to a nursing home. In my experience, I've seen many people thought to be unable to express themselves make their thoughts known, loud, and clear, when motivated by anger or other extreme emotion.

In the aftermath of this scenario, the nurse who accompanied the group on the field trip documented the resident's reaction as behavior in need of psychiatric assessment. I didn't see it the same way.

From my empathetic perspective, she was expressing an opinion and exercising her right as an independent adult to not get off the bus. Her perception of what was happening was obviously based in her memory of a similar situation. Perhaps she was thinking this was a city bus dropping her off at her home, and she didn't remember that the nursing home had been her home for the past three years.

Remove the nursing home residency and the dementia. None of us would get off the bus in that scenario if it wasn't our usual or expected stop. If the person has a diagnosis of mental illness underlying the dementia, the reaction might be laced with some paranoia about being taken to a nursing home against her will.

There are countless nursing home residents who will tell you how they were forced or tricked into coming to the nursing home by their family or a trusted advisor. No one dreams of living under someone else's rule. Nursing home placement is generally not the individual's decision. The decision is often made following a health related crisis by family members and medical professionals. Few nursing home residents actually want to be there.

The complication of dementia does make it more difficult to understand the motivation for the reaction, but analyzed in the way

I've described changes everything. If you put an average adult who lives in a society that values free movement and privacy above everything, the transition to the nursing home is bound to trigger extreme emotion.

In most cases, the caregiving staff is unprepared to respond appropriately to the anguish, depression, and general disgust that impacts the person confined to the nursing home environment. While the long-term care industry has done well to improve medical care, addressing behavioral health issues successfully remains an area in need of attention.

In fact, many people with dementia attempt to leave to go home or to find a family member they are searching for in the first few days of admission. For this reason, many facilities utilize an electronic system to monitor the whereabouts of residents determined to be at risk for elopement.

The electronic device generally takes the form of a bracelet or wristwatch that the person is unable to remove without assistance. In some cases, the device is attached to the person's ankle instead of their wrist in an effort to diminish attention to the device.

In my experience, the person wearing the device eventually learns that it will sound if he/she attempts to leave a defined area so many people are focused on trying to remove it. I liken it to being in survival mode. Despite the dementia or other cognitive deficit, the individual is still able to find a way out.

In V's case, he refused to wear the device and removed it each time it was applied, usually with a nail clipper he'd stolen from the nurses' station. He could be very charming, distracting the nurse or clerk behind the station while he secretly pocketed the nail clipper.

On the day he left, he actually walked out the front door of the home with a group of visitors. Since he'd rid himself of the monitoring bracelet, again, he left undetected.

When he was returned to the facility, I went to interview him about his experience and what motivated him to leave. In my role, I am often asked to help staff understand and develop successful, personalized responses to mood and behavior. Interviewing residents has become a routine part of my work, helping me to improve my understanding of what makes people tick and my ability to translate that understanding into effective remedies.

V told me he left the facility because he had to go to work. "If I don't work, I don't get paid, lady, you know?" Yes, I know. "What kind of work do you do?" I asked. He's a printer. He started the job in 1972, so he thinks he's had the job for about two years now.

Remember that he has a brain injury. His answer to my question helps me to understand where his thinking is at the moment. To avoid a negative interaction, it becomes necessary to understand the person's reality and to validate that reality rather than challenge it.[6] Doing so will not only avoid conflict but help to build a trusting relationship between the resident and caregiver.

I took a printing class in high school in the 1970s, so I was familiar with how printing was accomplished before computers. I asked him if he organized his letters in a drawer, and he said, "Yes, that's what I do!"

The next day, I approached him with a printer's drawer that I'd fashioned out of a box. It had a compartment for every letter, just like the drawer he was familiar with. I explained that I could use his help sorting the letters I had in another box.

He reminded me that he was going home soon and would not be able to help for long. I thanked him for whatever assistance he could give me in the time he was there, and he accepted. He sat down and didn't move again for more than ninety minutes while he worked.

Over the next few days, I made the task a little more difficult so that it would take him longer to complete it. I asked him to not only sort the letters but organize the letters for words I'd written down. He took great pride in doing this work, and soon his desire to leave the environment began to wane.

He eventually asked if he was going to be paid for his work. It made sense that he would want to be compensated for his work. I explained that he would be compensated in facility currency, also known as a

---

[6] Feil, Naomi, *The Validation Breakthrough: Simple Techniques for Communicating with People with Alzheimer's and Other Dementias, Third Edition.*

token economy. The facility dollars are numbered to minimize the incentive for theft. The numbered dollars cannot be traded or sold and must be redeemed only by the person who earned it.

He accepted the facility currency, later asking what he could buy with these dollars. I asked him what he would like to buy, and he responded, "Beer and pizza!" So, at the end of the week, he exchanged his facility currency for pizza and a frosty mug of beer.

The beer contained no alcohol, but recognizing that he could read and process what he was reading, I did not serve the beer in the bottle that clearly stated it was non-alcoholic beer. Instead, I served him an overflowing, frozen mug of beer. How delightful!

His eyes and his grin widened. He said, "Wow, that's a lot of beer!" "You earned it, enjoy!" I replied. He not only enjoyed his pizza and beer but later confessed to getting a little "buzz" from the beer. He said it did him good. I asked if he enjoyed his work. He did. He looked forward to working and reaping his reward. He liked being a man who is able to live the way he prefers to live.

Early in my career, I met two people with dementia who helped me understand that validating thoughts rather than challenging them was the way to go. At that time, Alzheimer's disease was not yet fully understood, so what I now know was Alzheimer's was diagnosed as a variety of cognitive disorders.

I didn't know anything about "therapy," and there was no one there to teach me, so I did what seemed reasonable. In most cases, I must confess, reasonable was equal to "stopped-the-screaming," whatever that might be. I learned a lot through trial and error. I also learned that you have to think differently, creatively, and know who you're talking to.

L was a lovely, blissfully confused lady of eighty-eight who would come to the activity room every evening around four thirty to prepare dinner for her husband. The activity room was equipped with a kitchenette, fueling L's perception that this was her kitchen.

The first time she explained to me that she had to cook dinner because her husband would be home soon, I didn't know how to respond. I knew, of course, that she wasn't thinking clearly, but I didn't understand the depth of the problem.

So, for lack of a better solution, I began asking questions about her husband. I asked his name, where he worked, and how they'd met. As the conversation continued, she stopped looking in the refrigerator and opening the oven door and sat down.

She began talking about how she met him and appeared to take great delight in retelling the story. The more she tried to express her feelings, often leaning back in her chair, hands gently crossed over her heart as she remembered and shared those memories with me, the calmer she became. Again, there was some word salad[7] thrown in, but her thinking became clearer the longer we talked.

As she finished her story of their wedding and the children they'd raised and the trip to Italy for their thirtieth anniversary, she told me that her husband had passed away. It took some time for her to remember this sad fact, but she finally did. Then, she got up, kissed the top of my head, and said she was sorry for taking so much of my time.

She continued to come every afternoon to fix her husband's dinner. I started involving her in simple food activity—icing cupcakes, cleaning string beans—and we would talk. I learned a great deal about her and the people in her life in those conversations.

One winter morning, as I was driving to work, I saw *L* walking down the sidewalk in her hospital gown. Barefoot, without her eyeglasses, and with the open back of her gown flapping in the frigid air. She looked lost and frightened.

I pulled over and rolled down the passenger's side window as I yelled to her, "*L*! Where are you going without your shoes and your coat? It's freezing out here. Everyone is worried about you." She looked down at her feet and then at me, "Yes, I'm cold. I'm very cold." I called out her husband's name, telling her he was worried and sent me to find her.

"Get in the car, and I'll take you home," I told her. I know now that being able to talk to her in familiar language, using names of people

---

[7] http://www.lbda.org/node/362.

she recognized was what worked to gain the trust of someone who otherwise wouldn't know you.

Being prepared to introduce any one of the many memories she's shared would help me to be familiar and safe despite her having no real memory of who I am or how she knows me. I knew her, and I knew her memories and could use those memories to be familiar now. It is this depth of knowledge that most caregivers lack, making it near impossible for most to really divert a confused, agitated, or otherwise distressed person's attention.

Today in my teaching, I encourage caregivers to document the memories shared by someone with dementia so they can remind them in detail of people and events when they no longer remember. Talking and recording memories is an effective and satisfying individualized activity for anyone but particularly therapeutic for someone with dementia.

J was a tall, distinguished-looking man of eighty-seven. He had a full head of silver hair that would get wavy if allowed to grow a little long. He wore wire-rimmed eyeglasses, often forgetting they were on his nose. "Where are my dang glasses? Did you take them?" he'd ask while peering at you through the very glasses he was looking for.

He was an engineer, described by his family as all work and no play. When he did take time to relax, he enjoyed listening to light, classical music. Piano music was his favorite. He also had an unusual skill—he could fashion animals out of pipe cleaners.

His son said he liked to work on his hobby late into the evening in his study. He said it helped him think, especially when the house was quiet. He'd created some very detailed animals, often giving them to his children when he was a younger man.

The person the caregivers in the facility came to know was not a kind or gentle soul. He was a very confused, impatient, agitated man who was difficult to satisfy and rude to the staff. In the days before I met him, his behavior had escalated to almost non-stop yelling and cursing. At that time, the only things known to calm him were a snack and medication.

He could be engaged in direct conversation for short periods if the atmosphere was quiet. I took the opportunity one afternoon to sit and talk with him. I asked how he was feeling, and he said he was fine. I asked if there was anything special he'd like to do. Before he could respond, I went on to tell him how his family had told me about his love of piano music and about his hobby of making animals out of pipe cleaners.

I referred several times to his son by name, chatting away, turning on the piano music, and offering him pipe cleaners and encouraging him to show me how he makes the animals. He started screaming at me and calling me stupid and some other words he'd made up on the spot in his anger! He made an attempt to stand up and, angered by the reality of his seatbelt, kept yelling, "I don't know! I don't know!" and rattling the buckle of the seatbelt.

His response frightened me. I would learn through these trial periods that he didn't like to listen to music and create pipe cleaner animals at the same time. He liked quiet and needed an environment that would let him concentrate when he was working on his animals. In his dementia, concentrating became increasingly difficult. Quiet helped him focus.

I would also learn that giving too much direction at one time was overwhelming. Some days later, left alone at the table in the quiet recreation room, he began to create his pipe cleaner animals. I had placed a large pile of pipe cleaners on the table and left him alone to "think." He stopped screaming.

We developed a daily activity plan for him that allowed him to spend his time in a quiet place. In the past, he'd been seated in the big, noisy dayroom, filled with other residents. The television would be on. The radio in the dayroom would be playing loudly to be heard over the piped in music playing overhead. Staff was talking even louder in an effort to hear each other over the other noise. After several hours in this environment—if any of us could even last a few hours—anyone would want to scream.

J never remembered making his animals. If you asked him to make one, he'd tell you he didn't know how. When you tried to convince him that he did know how and that he'd made them in the past, he'd start yelling, calling you a "doggone fibber!"

It was OK that he didn't remember. As long as his hands remembered how to do the task, he was able to make his animals, even if his brain wasn't fully engaged. A 2011 article addressing memory and communication explains how the motor component of an activity makes it possible for people like *J* to be able to do something, even if they don't remember that they can do it:

> The motor component of a task is believed to make it more memorable, as it enriches the **encoding experience** and often involves the manipulation of concrete objects. There is further evidence that people with dementia are able to maintain or relearn activities of daily living (e.g., setting the table, preparing a meal) with appropriate environmental support and active regular practice.[8]

I've met many other people like *J* whose hands could do things they no longer remembered they could do. This is especially true of a person who played a musical instrument, someone who quilted or did needlework, or someone whose former occupation required a repetitive action. Like assembly work in a factory.

In replicating the task, these people are generally able to do some rote activity and find satisfaction in the structure and repetition of it. No matter what the task is, it is perceived as purposeful *work* and when it's done, it feels good.

What Do I Do Now, Nurse?

Meaningful activity, in my mind, is something that I really want to do, something I look forward to, something I plan for, and often,

---

[8] Pachana, Nancy, "Memory and Communication Support in Dementia: Research-Based Strategies For Caregivers," Cambridge University Press: Jan 1, 2011.

something I share with people I enjoy being with. In some cases, the things I find meaningful help to define who I am.

I think of myself as a musician first because music has always been central to my quality of life. In addition to being a musician, I enjoy drawing and painting, cooking, baking, pottery, gardening, theater, concerts, traveling, hosting dinner parties, and so many other things. I am multifaceted, as are you, and every dependent person I've ever met.

In preparation for a seminar for activity professionals I was presenting at, I researched activity schedules from long-term care facilities around the country. According to these monthly calendars, the average resident of a nursing home or assisted living facility will drink coffee as a meaningful activity twelve to fifteen times a week.

You're probably thinking drinking coffee sounds like a pretty good thing. The truth of the matter is that the coffee in most of these facilities is not the same as the coffee you might have at home or pick up at the local coffee boutique. In a culture rumored to be addicted to coffee, having coffee that isn't made the way you like it will not be fun or meaningful.

What passes for meaningful activity in most long-term care environments is a far cry from what you or I would really do. While I understand that some dependent people are regressing or have a special need that requires the activity be modified, much of the activity directed at those with dementia or other special needs infantilize the population and can be less than therapeutic.

There are those social activities that more capable residents engage in, like games, luncheons, parties, and field trips. In my interviews, even the most alert and capable mourn the loss of meaningful work. Social activities are good, they'll tell you, but they'd like something more challenging, more intellectually stimulating.

Considering the staggering numbers of people who have dementia, the numbers who can appreciate what is offered without accommodation for their declining understanding and communication will shrink. It is common for only certain residents to be invited to a group or event. Those who challenge the activity staff because they are declining and difficult to engage are usually left behind.

It is also common for the activity staff to be undereducated or underexposed to the places, people, and events that will stimulate the memory of the residents they are providing programming for. There is no education requirement for activity staff beyond the mandatory education in residents' rights, abuse prevention, and safety required for all staff.

Some years ago, the Centers for Medicare and Medicaid conducted a large-scale study of nursing home residents in New York State regarding their thoughts on what constitutes quality of life and meaningful activity. The study found that residents:

- Assigned priority to dignity
- Identified the two main components of dignity as independence and positive self-image
- Favor activities that amount to something, such as those that produce or teach something, activities using skills from residents' former work, religious activities, and activities that contribute to the nursing home.
- Indicated that a lack of appropriate activities contributes to having no sense of purpose
- Want a variety of activities, including those that are not childish, require thinking, are gender-specific, produce something useful, relate to previous work of residents, allow for socializing with visitors and participating in community events, and are physically active.

The report stated that residents not only discussed particular activities that gave them a sense of purpose but also indicated that a lack of appropriate activities contributes to having no sense of purpose. Residents rarely mentioned participating in activities as a way to just keep busy or just to socialize. The relevance of the activities to the residents' lives must be considered.

The study also found that the above concepts were relevant to both interviewable and non-interviewable residents. Researchers observed that non-interviewable residents appeared "happier" and "less agitated" in homes with many planned activities for them.[9]

Developing Person-Centered, Meaningful Activity

Barring very severe disability or late-stage cognitive deficit, the vast majority of residents prefer a day filled with purposeful work. I have interviewed thousands of residents in my years as a consultant and observed or worked with many others in a host of social and structured activity settings—most would rather work and accomplish something than sit passively while someone else does something to entertain them.

I had the good fortune to share an office with the social workers and occupational and physical therapists in one of my early nursing homes. It was through that exposure that I learned what made an activity therapeutic physically or cognitively and what had to be done to make it therapeutic intellectually and emotionally.

In 1991, I hired Terrence Hicks to work as an activity leader in the recreation department I managed in a local nursing home. Like many of the people I hired at that time, he was not experienced, but he was in college and interested in learning.

Today, Terrence is an occupational therapist at a prominent hospital in New York City. Throughout our friendship, we have had many conversations about helping those we care for have a better life experience. We agree that boredom and a lack of purposeful activity will not only negatively impact an individual's mood and reactions but contribute significantly to his/her ability to communicate and function successfully in the world.

Over the years, Terrence and I have discussed activities on many levels. What is known today as activity or recreation therapy evolved out of OT in the early 1970s. Having worked in both occupational and

---

[9] CMS State Operations Manual, Appendix PP, F248 Activities—Interpretive Guidelines.

recreation therapy, Terrence has a perspective on the subject that is unique to his experience.

In the next passage, Terrence explains the relationship between therapeutic, meaningful activity and quality of life.

Central to the lives of all human beings are occupations. Occupations are how we spend or occupy our time in daily life. This is vital to mental and physical health, and happiness and success as individuals despite the presence of disease or disability. Occupational therapy is rooted in promoting its recipients to participate in meaningful occupations and activities to achieve a productive and healthy life and to maximize a person's quality of life.

Quality of life refers to the general well-being of people from all walks of life. Quality of life can be rich as observed in those who are able to freely pursue self-care, hobbies, employment, and life roles, or quality of life can be poor as observed in those who lack opportunity to pursue or participate in desired activities.

Many years ago, in a facility where I worked, I frequently saw well-dressed residents who looked like they had a place to go or something to do, but they ended up sitting in wheelchairs in the hallways staring into space or wandering the hallways aimlessly. The idea that common, everyday activities can be utilized therapeutically is simple, clever, and underrated. During the day-to-day grind in "dealing" with residents who may have complex medical, psychological, or social needs, we may "overthink" our intervention options.

You may ask a resident what is it that they need or want to do. Often, they do not know or cannot clearly express their desires if they have any idea of them at all. In my experience, many of the people I work with are not able to spontaneously verbalize these things. It takes time and skilled observation of your residents to find these answers. You may mutually achieve this information.

There are many people who may be incapacitated, disabled, or otherwise impaired who led very productive lives prior to this onset and now may "act out" or become depressed because of their dependency. This maladaptive behavior is unproductive and can lead to other issues both clinical and administrative in health care settings.

While it is important for these residents to receive the therapy expected in a medical model, there is opportunity for occupational and activity therapists to work collaboratively to highlight the importance of meaningful activities to improve health outcomes, patient care, and ultimately, patient satisfaction.

The Activity Workshop

While working in one of my first nursing homes in Ohio, I learned about sheltered workshops. These were occupationally based, therapeutic, community programs in which adults with developmental or emotional disabilities would engage in piece-work.

Projects in these workshops might involve assembling or packing items for local organizations or business owners. Other projects designed for those with less skill might involve "busy work," such as sorting, counting, or matching activities. The people working in these programs were paid a small stipend each week for their work.

For those who attended the workshop, going to work was generally a very important part of their life. No matter how someone else might view the "job," those residents I worked with enjoyed being productive, having responsibility, and contributing something seen as important. There's no denying that the stipend was an added incentive, but I believe the structure, routine, familiarity, and potential to succeed every day had a lot to do with it, too.

I continue to encourage the development of this model over the large group activities that are common to nursing homes, assisted living, and adult daycare environments. Residents are offered entertainment-based activity for brief periods of time in between the various types of care being provided. There is a start-and-stop rhythm to the day that is both exhausting and tedious. The workshop model provides for a more normal pattern of successive activities that are linked together rather than conducted as distinct parts.

In the current environmental design, residents have brief periods of busy activity, such as during a meal, or a bath, or a bingo game, followed by longer periods of sitting idle. Many residents fall asleep during these interludes, only to be startled awake by the caregiver at the beginning of the next task.

It is common to see residents awakened out of sound sleep only to find a spoon full of food being pushed into their mouth before they can get their bearings. When the startled resident pushes the caregiver's hand away in confusion, the action will be interpreted as being aggressive or resistive, rather than as a reasonable response to not understanding what's going on.

The workshop allows for a structured day to flow from one type of activity to another without the common stopping and starting that complicates residents' reactions to so many environments. Each resident is offered a task that has been developed specific to the resident's former occupation or lifestyle or a simplified, rote task designed to engage and provide physical and sensory stimulation.

Occupationally based tasks are most successful when the tools of the trade are utilized over commercial items. Someone who was once a banker might be engaged in counting money or adding numbers. A former clerical worker might find pleasure in stuffing or stamping envelopes.

One former secretary I met enjoyed sorting the large, vinyl-covered paperclips by color into baby food jars. In her mind, she was simply organizing the clips and happy to do it. It gave her a sense of accomplishment.

In some cases, residents are invited to help accomplish something for someone else. I often explain to a resident I want to engage that what they will be helping me do will benefit another resident who is not as well as the resident who is being asked to help. I believe it is in the charity of helping another that the motivation to do whatever is asked is accepted.

Residents who are unable to engage in domestic or occupational tasks might benefit from music or audio recordings offered to them via an iPod or Walkman. If the resident's family is willing to record an audio reminiscence recording of a memorable event or other stories the resident's memory might be stimulated by, the recordings can be an invaluable intervention. The familiarity of the voice and the content of the memory being shared is often a soothing intervention for those with dementia.

The workshop model allows for many residents to occupy a shared environment but enjoy an individualized activity that is appealing. The environment of the workshop is maintained as quiet and calm, allowing people to better concentrate and removing some of the common triggers to negative behavior like noise and excessive activity. Maintaining a quiet, calm, comfortable, work environment will be a key factor in sustaining the residents' tolerance for that environment.

Residents who can be engaged in tasks but who react poorly to being in the large group can be offered that task in another setting. Allowing residents who appear to prefer smaller groups or being alone to work apart from the group will often solve other mood and response issues.

Television and music should be utilized sparingly, as there are few large groups of people in any environment who will share interest in a particular television show or music genre. Most adults have very specific viewing and listening preferences that cannot be enjoyed in such a diverse group. Add to the sheer numbers the fact that the noise and excessive activity in the environment will prevent the residents from even hearing the television or music, and the need for better organization and control is clear.

Oversight and supervision of the resident population is accomplished currently by stationing a CNA or other caregiver in the common area to watch the residents. During these watching times, there is generally no activity offered. The television or music might be on but neither is directed to any specific interest. Most often, the television is tuned to the program the caregiver assigned to supervision wants to watch.

This ritual of watching could easily give way to a more mature and common manner of providing for the safety of the residents if there was an expectation that every caregiver would focus attention on making sure the resident's day is structured and purposeful. As it now stands, most organizations structure a day according to the needs and timetables of the worker, not the resident.

"Culture change" is the common name given to the national movement for the transformation of older adult services, based on person-directed values and practices where the voices of elders and those working with them are considered and respected. Core, person-directed values are choice, dignity, respect, self-determination, and purposeful living.[10]

To achieve and sustain the kind of quality living environment on which the culture change movement is built, the focus of caregivers must shift from getting the task done to achieving the best outcome for the resident every day. That will only happen when there are sufficient numbers of well-trained, appropriately supervised, and supported staff functioning in an environment that is organized, consistent, comfortable, and always looking for new and superior methods of satisfying the people who have no choice but to live there.

What Constitutes Homelike for the Dependent Person?

The personalized care ideal focuses on creating an environment that is homelike for the resident. In a population as diverse as the long-term

---

[10] http://www.pioneernetwork.net/CultureChange/.

care community, finding a common description of what is homelike will be a challenge.

Based on the experiences I've had over the course of my career, I would venture to say that the definition of homelike is as personal as the defining criteria for an individual's quality of life. The one-size-fits-all environment gives way to people feeling lost in the shuffle and bitter in the face of what many consider to be captivity.

A typical response to being overlooked would be to utilize "attention-getting behavior," like complaining to the manager or writing a bad review of the company on the Internet. In the nursing home environment, complaining is often seen as an act requiring psychiatric evaluation.

Based on the responses to many interviews on what constitutes a satisfying environment, two important ingredients for creating a satisfying, homelike environment are control and privacy, both of which are lost when you cross the threshold of an institutionalized community. Once there, you follow the rules, abide by the restrictions that are placed on you by the people caring for you, and learn to assimilate as best you can for the time you are there.

There are many things that could be done to increase the control and privacy available to the people living in the institutional community. One wonderful change would be allowing people to sit apart from the group. That large, crowded, noisy, uncomfortable dayroom is no place to spend your twilight years or the rest of your long life, if you are unlucky enough to be dependent but not old.

Many of the caregivers that I've spoken with will tell you that corralling people in one room is the only efficient way to prevent something bad from happening to any of them. What they fail to realize is that they are creating a hotbed of unrest and dissatisfaction, a climate that is sure to override whatever benefit they feel they are getting from this method of supervision. Causing people to remain sitting still for long periods of time with nothing interesting to do is the worst approach to keeping them safe and happy.

The workshop model is one alternative, finding more creative ways to allow people to disperse and still be safe would be another. I have observed that residents who are truly engaged in an activity that interests and challenges them are not interested in doing the things that generally put them at risk for harm, like ambulating without assistance or eloping.

One client facility implemented a system of ambulatory or "walking" supervision. This approach allows residents to remain in their rooms or in smaller groups while still receiving the oversight needed to maintain a safe environment.

In this model, the CNA who would normally be assigned to a thirty-minute stationary supervision of the big, common room instead patrols the unit, observing residents in their preferred setting. Each participating CNA documents the whereabouts of each resident as he/she makes rounds and indicates what the resident was doing at the time of the observation on a form designed for this purpose.

Residents are then able to take a nap, watch a favorite show on television, listen to music that appeals to them, and simply have the freedom and choice to do as they please. There will always be those who require more direct supervision, however, the formula of the workshop model, coupled with walking supervision, proves a viable alternative to the large, annoying group.

Longtime friend, mentor, and colleague, Patricia Brown, RN, offers her thoughts on what the transition to long-term care must feel like for the resident. She echoes the feelings of countless other caregivers I've spoken with on the need for more human contact in dependent communities. She understands both clinically and personally the impact of positive, nurturing relationships and purposeful living on the quality of a life or of a living environment.

> When I think about residents in the nursing home setting, I think about the transition from a life of independence to total dependence. Just think of the transition coming from your own home to sharing a room with a total stranger, from browsing a look in the refrigerator to waiting for someone to offer food or beverage.

As a registered nurse for many years, I have seen dramatic changes in healthcare, particularly in long-term care. The most skilled level of nursing professional spends most of the day knee-deep in paperwork. Remember, if it's not written, it is not done. We hear that so often.

Just think about this scenario: It is 7:00 p.m. The nurse on the unit is a licensed practical nurse who is responsible for forty residents. The nurse needs to administer medication and treatments, answer the phone, call physicians, interact with families, respond to emergencies, and a thousand other things.

This nurse has several CNAs assigned to the unit. They each have an assignment that includes feeding, toileting, comfort care, ambulation, range of motion exercise, and a thousand other things to accomplish relative to the care of their assigned residents. I am getting tired just thinking about how exhausting this evening will be.

The day may start out well, but by 7:00 p.m., residents become tired and cranky, and Sundowning [11] behavior begins. They may not have liked the dinner meal. Their families have gone home. Now, at the busiest time of the evening, moods and behavior become more concerning. Residents become agitated, more verbally and physically aggressive, and more weepy and unhappy.

Again, she reminds us that there are not enough hands to achieve the kind of person-centered care we aspire to. In the circumstance of too many needs and not enough human resources that she has described, the popular remedy is often a call to the physician for medication.

---

[11] People with Alzheimer's and dementia may have problems sleeping or increases in behavioral problems that begin at dusk and last into the night, known as Sundowning syndrome: http://www.alz.org/care/alzheimers-dementia-sleep-issues-sundowning.asp.

For many, the remedy is all about more resources. If the additional hands recruited are not properly educated and trained, more will not equal improved. The successful remedy relies on six key ingredients:

1. Excellent clinical care and treatment;
2. An educated, well-trained, empathetic staff;
3. A physical environment that is not only clean, safe, and comfortable but provides for the privacy and control of every individual to the extent possible;
4. An ambiance that is warm, friendly, familiar, and supportive of every individual enjoying a quality of life that is satisfying;
5. A purposeful daily routine of meaningful social and diversionary activities that are designed with the individual in mind; and
6. Food that is satisfying, surprising, and something to anticipate and enjoy.

It has been my experience that more staff is not always the answer. There continue to be facilities that have staffing levels that are more generous than others. The level of understanding and personalized care does not increase simply by hiring more people.

For example, in one facility, a new position was created to supplement the CNAs working on the unit. These new workers were to assist with meals, activities, transporting residents, and other general duties in the environment.

Within a month of hire, six of the eight new staff hired had resigned. The feedback from the departing workers indicated that there was a lack of real orientation and supervision for these workers, putting them in the position to work independently in an environment and with people they really knew nothing about.

Too few facilities invest in the type of education and staff support that is really necessary to ensure quality is maintained on all levels. The tough financial climate has caused long-term care facilities to consolidate positions and pare down departments in an effort to balance the budget. Unfortunately, some of those first to go are those who provide education and oversight to the staff.

Without a consistent educator who enjoys teaching and is success-ful at motivating staff to value education, the facility will fall victim time and again to human error and tragedy that is caused by ignorance or lack of experience. In reviewing deficiency citations resulting from facility inspections by the state health department, the cause can often be traced back to staff who should have had knowledge or should have acted but didn't.

Some years ago, I was one of a team of consultants involved in a sex-ual assault case. Following a very serious deficiency citation from the health department, my colleagues and I were retained to assist the facility in achieving their corrective plan. Depending on the scope and severity of the problem(s) identified, a facility is sometimes required to hire consultants to oversee the repair of staff education practices and facility policies relative to the errors made.

The findings in this case involved a female resident with Alzheimer's dementia who was being routinely assaulted sexually by a male staff member. The resident's neighbor across the corridor witnessed this behavior on many occasions over a period of months. She told a number of staff, including nursing and social service department managers, about what she was seeing, but no one acted to investigate.

In the end, the neighbor across the corridor reported the abuse to the health department, and an investigation ensued. There was no arrest in the case because both the victim and the reporting wit-ness had a diagnosis of dementia. The victim had no ability to com-municate effectively due to her declining cognition. The neighbor was in an earlier stage of her dementia but was still considered unreliable.

The perpetrator was terminated from his position. The victim and her neighbor continued to reside in the facility and receive care as they had before the incident.

During a later conversation with some of the staff who had heard about the abuse but not acted to investigate the allegation, most said they didn't respond because the accused staff member "didn't look like someone who would do something like that." The other reason offered was that both the victim and the neighbor were confused.

With better education, those same staff members would have known that every accusation needs to be investigated, even those reported by residents with a dementia diagnosis, if only to verify if its truth or fantasy. In the absence of any investigation, events like this sexual assault that lasted months longer than it should have will continue to happen.

There are countless tragedies occurring every day due to declining numbers of caregivers, poor education and oversight of the staff, and the growing despair throughout the industry over the increasingly difficult operational climate. The realities of our national healthcare crisis have significantly impacted long-term care.

The changes that are yet to come as Medicare and Medicaid services become part of managed care networks will further impact the morale of long-term care providers. The willingness and motivation to look beyond minimum compliance to creating an environment of care that is truly livable will also decline.

five

A Recipe for Improving Quality of Life in Long-Term Care

"The purpose of life is to live it, to taste experience to the utmost, to reach out eagerly and without fear for newer and richer experience."

—*Eleanor Roosevelt*

Creating a truly livable environment that promotes optimum quality of life despite challenges requires a deeper commitment to know the people being cared for—what they've experienced and sacrificed, how they've lived, and what they hope for now. Helping someone achieve a quality of life that sustains them requires introspection and consideration of the question, "What would I want if I were the one being cared for?"

All too often, the institutional environment takes on a warehouse-like ambiance, where keeping people clean, dry, and well-fed takes precedence over keeping them happy and engaged in living. There are a multitude of regulations requiring that people be afforded all of those things adults value—privacy, dignity, respect, safety, choice—yet there is a great divide between what is expected, or even mandated, and what is actually provided.

Annual inspections motivate some deeper thinking on these issues, but the impact is rarely lasting. Insiders would describe the gearing up and winding down cycle associated with annual inspections as everyone on their toes and alert to issues in need of attention until inspection is over. While they are randomly and confidentially scheduled, there is still some predictability to the inspection system. For the periods immediately preceding and following an annual inspection, care, service, and attention to detail are heightened.

In the remaining six or seven months of the year, much of the attention turns to the struggle of the staff to accomplish the work with the resources they have or to address challenging residents without education or resources or to manage office politics or to be swallowed up by the personal challenges that impact so many of the staff. Residents and their ongoing needs become business as usual, until the next time something shakes up the status quo.

There are many, many dedicated and compassionate professionals in long-term care who have grown weary of swimming upstream. Too many are stranded in organizations that have lost their way, fighting an uphill battle every day to accomplish the most basic level of care. A good number are leaving the field, opting to explore a new occupation, rather than navigate the increasingly difficult world of long-term care.

There is no one, ultimate plan to resolve all of the challenges impacting the quality of life for people living dependently in long-term care environments. What will work is careful selection and education of the staff, capable leadership and oversight, and systems that focus staff attention on accommodating the needs of the people they are caring for over their own needs.

Changing the thinking of the people providing the care is preferable to adding more undereducated, poorly supervised bodies to the mix. The caregiving staff must take a genuine interest in the people they are caring for. That will only happen when it is modeled behavior, an expectation, a requirement of continued employment, and held as the most significant of facility values.

It would help a great deal if there were more acknowledgement and recognition of a difficult job done well from those who direct these communities. With fewer hands than ever before, it is vital that those who remain to do the hard work are valued and supported. Greater efforts should be made to shrink the labor/management divide.

I do not expect that the numbers of hands available to care will increase in the future. I do expect that our systems and strategies for managing the complicated, human needs of many will have to change by sheer necessity. How well an organization weathers those changes will depend on how willing the staff is to accept that change must come. They will also be wise to recognize the benefit of paying attention to detail.

Improve the coffee. Offer residents the opportunity to enjoy a hot, frothy cup of cappuccino occasionally, or a little French vanilla creamer, or at least serve whatever coffee you have while it's still hot.

Quiet the noise. Make it a capital offense to be unnecessarily noisy in the environment. Just as there are fines in New York City for honking your car horn, there should be fines in long-term care facilities for noise violations perpetrated by the staff.

Lose the attitude. Do everything possible, including ridding your facility of staff who are hopelessly rude and insensitive, to cultivate a staff that is mature and respectful of their clientele and each other.

Mature the activity. Expect and support programming that is designed to promote cognitive, psychosocial, and functional health and to help the individual maintain the highest degree of personal quality and satisfaction.

Breed Empathy. Talk everyday about the importance of seeing the world through the eyes of the one being care for. Challenge every caregiver to recognize the individuality of each resident, and tailor care to meet those specific needs.

I believe the future of quality long-term care relies on recognizing that the body does not operate separate from the mind and spirit. Holistic care is the key to quality of life. Caregivers need to be prepared to understand and heal the whole person, not just the physical being.

The most important ingredients to a quality existence are people to care for and about and something interesting and meaningful to work toward. Where there is better education, deeper assessment and understanding of the individual and an environment that values creativity, common sense, and attention to detail, an improved quality of life is in reach.

34221451R00052

Made in the USA
Middletown, DE
12 August 2016